If you love it
If you don't –

CHOICE MATTERS

Paul and Barbara Gerhardt

PAUL AND BARBARA
GERHARDT

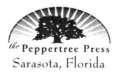

the **Peppertree Press**
Sarasota, Florida

For information regarding permission,
call 941-922-2662 or contact us at our website:
www.peppertreepublishing.com or write to:
the Peppertree Press, LLC.
Attention: Publisher
1269 First Street, Suite 7
Sarasota, Florida 34236

ISBN: 978-1-936343-57-7

Library of Congress Number: 2010942583

Printed in the U.S.A.

Printed January 2011

This book is dedicated to all sincere people who want to make this country and world a better place to live and who choose to be a part of the solution and not a part of the problem.

INTRODUCTION

This is a book about choice. It is about the choices we can make and the choices we would like to make, but which are forbidden to us. The choices are not only personal, but societal, as well. This book takes the position that freedom to choose is important. It is essential to ultimate happiness and to a truly free and just society. True freedom means choice.

It is also a book full of personal opinions. They are the opinions of two people, Barbara and Paul, who have spent most of their lives together, loving, caring, bitching, moaning, questioning, discussing, and trying to find the answers to some of the vexing problems we face in our society. We have not attempted to footnote references, but refer to some sources within the text. Most of the factual information to which we refer is common knowledge or readily accessible on the internet. Again, these are personal opinions which voice our frustrations and concerns and are expressed in the hope that they will generate more thought and discussions on the various topics we have chosen to tackle. Perhaps, by expressing our personal observations and opinions on these subjects, we will be a catalyst for change and a wider recognition that freedom means choice and, therefore, CHOICE MATTERS.

TABLE OF CONTENTS

PERSONAL REFLECTIONS

Looking in the mirror, what do we see? We see an image of our bodily self. Good or bad, it is what we have to walk around in and what we present for the world to see. There are things which we do to try to project a better image, but the thing which costs the least and does the most is a smile, and "putting one on" actually will affect our moods in a positive way. There are many things we can do to improve our "looks" beyond putting on a smile, but they can be costly and time-consuming. If we have been diligent in brushing and flossing our teeth, we may still have them, but are they crooked or white enough? We can get them straightened, whitened, or capped if that will make us feel better, but that is our choice - if we can afford it.

Barbara:

At seventy plus, the face I see looking back at me could use lots of help, especially when I peruse any of the many glamour magazines which tempt me when I stand in line at the grocery store, but I have not yet decided to have it lifted, tucked, or filled. I may, but not yet. That is my choice. Some twenty years ago, I perceived a very mean, frowning face peering at me and since I didn't feel mean and even a smile didn't seem to overcome the mean, saggy, baggy eyelid look, I did make the choice to have my upper eyelids "lifted". My plastic surgeon took pictures of the skin, fat, and muscle he removed from my upper lids and remarked that he had never seen such baggy eyelids on a fifty year old, but that my Scandinavian heritage was probably a contributing factor. Maybe it's the awful weather in those areas which makes folks frown and develop baggy eyelids. Who knows, but I felt and looked so much happier after the surgery. It was a good choice for me.

Physical appearance and health also have a definite effect on mental attitude and are, in part, affected by hereditary and environmental influences. How we all love to be a "victim" when something bad happens to us. No one likes to say, "It's my fault that I developed lung cancer". How much more satisfying to say, " Cigarettes caused my lung cancer" or, "All of those bad, fast-food restaurants caused my obesity". Each of us has choices every day which affect our health and appearance. We have become a nation of victims and our victim mentality has pushed the demand for government help and entitlements for people who could, by making better choices, be healthier, stronger, and work to support themselves and others. The old J.F. Kennedy slogan, "Ask not what your country can do for you, but what you can do for your country" has been reversed and has changed us from a nation of "can do" people to "poor me" people.

Barbara:
When I was diagnosed with breast cancer, I had to make choices regarding what treatment to accept. I was advised by my doctors, but ultimately had the last say, which is how it should be. Pathology reports turned out to back up the decision I made to go with a mastectomy, although that was not what the doctor was suggesting. When I was asked for advice regarding an unwanted pregnancy, I had choices about what to say. At the time abortion was illegal and unsafe. I was begged to help in ending a life of pain from an incurable disease, and I had a choice to make. Such help is still illegal in most states. How would you chose? Would you choose to obey the laws set up by the government or break the law?

ELEMENTS OF
CHOICE

When you think about all of the elements affecting choice, you realize how many there are and how different they may be in any varying situation. Choice, first and foremost, must be determined by common good, or at least be lawful and not cause harm to another person or society in general. Choice, also, is swayed by personal opinions and beliefs. Clearly, my personal right to swing my arm around is limited by the proximity of your nose. The biggest limiter of free choice is the government and its influence should be only in areas which are deemed to be common good concerns, not personal choice areas. The difference is not always easy to determine. The government has the right to tax us. Without taxation, we would not have roads, free public schools, social security, military and police protection, medical research, the FBI, the CIA, unemployment compensation, jails, or social welfare programs. Unfortunately, the power to tax and spend our money is directed by human beings, who are fallible, corruptible and, in some cases, downright dishonest, a fact which in turn mandates more costly controls.

The other major institutions which limit choice, through both institutional rules, as well as beliefs which are internalized by the members, are the religious institutions. These are our churches, synagogues, mosques, and other religious groups which are supported by voluntary members. The limitations on choice, which these religious institutions espouse, are accepted by each member on a voluntary basis. In most cases, people are not forced to join a religious group. Our constitution says that our government will not establish a religion or have any religious requirement for office. It seems our founding fathers did not establish a theocracy, but did not forbid the free practice of religion within the constraints of the law.

Some tenets of various faiths restrict choice for their members who accept these restrictions. It is their right to set up rules for the conduct of their members if they are not against governmental laws. Early Jewish laws were very restrictive. These laws applied to purity, food preparation and consumption, sacrifices, circumcision, unclean animals, leprosy, and sexual relationships. Their laws regarding childbirth were also definitely gender-biased. " When a woman gives birth and bears a male child, then she shall be unclean for seven days….and remain in the blood of her purification for thirty-three days, but if she bears a female child, she shall be unclean for two weeks and the days of her purification would be sixty-six days". The laws served to reflect the holiness of God, to keep Israel distinct from the "idolatrous" nations around them, and to help maintain physical health. Foods which were ruled unclean and were to be avoided included eels, shellfish, lobsters, crabs, oysters, rabbits, pigs, eagles, vultures, ravens, storks, herons, pelicans, cats, dogs, mice, etc, etc. Today some Jews still observe very restrictive food rules, but some do not, depending on the type or category of synagogue which they attend.

Catholics have fewer restrictions placed upon them, and Protestants even fewer. Restrictions are established by the church hierarchy. Both Catholic and Protestant groups espouse the Ten Commandments given to Moses on Mount Sinai, as well as strive to understand and follow the teachings of Jesus. All sorts of litigation has been initiated regarding the displaying of the Ten Commandments on government property or in government buildings and there are valid reasons to restrict such display to religious property.

The Catholic church has had specific restrictions instituted by male church leaders concerning sexuality, including bans on using contraceptives, which have had far-reaching consequences, and will be discussed later. These bans, if adhered to, greatly restrict the element of choice and mostly affect women.

WOMEN'S REPRODUCTIVE ISSUES

The most talked about and argued about reproductive issue is that of a woman's right of access to the medical procedure known as abortion. From Wikipedia the following gives insight into the much discussed Roe v. Wade decision. "Roe v. Wade, decided on January 22, 1973, was a landmark decision by the United States Supreme Court on the issue of abortion. The Court held that a woman's right to an abortion is determined by the stage of pregnancy, and that the state cannot prohibit abortion before viability. After viability, the state cannot prohibit abortion if abortion "is necessary, in appropriate medical judgment, for the preservation of the life or health of the mother" as defined in the companion case of Doe v. Bolton. The Court said that "viability" means potentially able to live outside the mother's womb, albeit with artificial aid. Viability is usually placed at about seven months (28 weeks), but may occur earlier, even at 24 weeks." The Court rested these conclusions on a constitutional right to privacy emanating from the Due Process Clause of the Fourteenth Amendment, also known as substantive due process. In disallowing many state and federal restrictions on abortion in the United States, Roe v. Wade prompted a national debate that continues today about issues including whether and to what extent abortion should be legal, who should decide the legality of abortion, what methods the Supreme Court should use in constitutional adjudication, and what the role should be of religious and moral views in the political sphere. Roe v. Wade reshaped national politics, dividing much of the nation into pro-choice and pro-life camps, while activating grass roots movements on both sides.

In section IX, The Court added that there were no legal grounds for factoring into this balancing test any right to life of the unborn fetus. The fetus would have such a right if it were defined as a legal person for purposes of the Fourteenth Amendment, but the original intent of the Constitution (up to the enactment of the Fourteenth Amendment in 1868), did not include protection of the unborn, according to the Court. The Court emphasized that its determination of whether a fetus can enjoy constitutional protection neither meant to reference, nor intervene in, the question of when life begins saying, "We need not resolve the difficult question of when life begins. When those trained in the respective disciplines of medicine, philosophy, and theology are unable to arrive at any consensus, the judiciary, at this point in the development of man's knowledge, is not in a position to speculate as to the answer."

In section X, the Court explained that the trimester of pregnancy is relevant to the weight of the factors in this balancing test. Thus, during the first and second trimesters, the state may only regulate the abortion procedure "in ways that are reasonably related to maternal health"; during the third trimester, the state can choose to restrict or proscribe abortion, as it sees fit when the fetus is viable ("except where it is necessary, in appropriate medical judgment, for the preservation of the life or health of the mother").

Since the Roe v. Wade decision, the right to have a safe legal abortion has been attacked, with pro-lifers attempting to gut Roe v. Wade a few procedures at a time. "Partial-birth abortion" laws, parental notification laws, and attempting to pass laws requiring a woman to pay for an unnecessary ultra-sound procedure before having an abortion are all calculated to keep women with unwanted pregnancies from a real choice in the matter. They are designed to stall 1st and 2nd trimester abortions until there is no chance for choice and the woman is stuck in a "forced pregnancy", with greater chance of death or complications of birth during the delivery than from an abortion, especially among the young. Ninety-nine percent of all abortions in 1997 occurred in the first twenty weeks. Most delays beyond that are now due to lack of providers nearby, poverty, teens in denial, fear of violence at provider clinics, the trauma of parental notification laws (especially if the parent is also the father), slow court proceedings, or learning from testing about severe fetal abnormalities. The partial-birth abortion ban would not stamp out infanticide, which is already illegal, but would cripple a woman and her doctor's rights to make a choice in a late stage of pregnancy, when they felt it necessary.

Abortion was well known and widely practiced in ancient times. No verse in the Bible supports or forbids abortion, however in Numbers, 5:12-28, it is prescribed in the case of a married woman who was impregnated by a man other than her husband and many non-scriptural writings explain how herbal abortifacients were used. The Puritans used abortion prior to the fetus being felt moving in the womb and it was a common practice until the mid-1800's when the churches began to make rules regarding its morality. The Bible says nothing regarding abortion to let us know whether or not it is right or wrong and there were legions of opportunities for the writers of the Bible to include a statement about it - whether to condone or forbid the known practice. The Bible is, therefore, a "pro-choice" book, leaving the decision up to the person or persons involved. If any of the commandments written regarding murder considered abortion murder, the writers did not include mention of this. Some women will feel that it is not the right thing for them, especially if internalized morality for them would not allow the procedure. Their choice has been made for them due to their belief. And that is fine. Some women will weigh the issues carefully before deciding. Choice will be based on feelings, perceptions, goals, and needs. Other women will make the choice to chose abortion easily based apparently on shallower reasons, but that should be their choice and a woman should not have to justify her decision to anyone. It is very important that one's opinion about the morality of abortion can and should be separate from his desire to make it illegal. The legal status of abortion has never affected the extent of its use, only its safety.

Paul: The following account tells of a choice made seventy-eight years ago. Abortion saved my life. A strange statement, isn't it? Let me explain. My father, who was born in 1899, was one of six children. My mother, who was born in 1905 was one of eleven. Neither came from wealthy families. One grandfather worked on the railroad and the other was a shoe salesman. So, the question arises: why did my grandparents have such large families when they were relatively poor? No, they weren't Catholic or Mormon. No, they were not wildly sexual - at least not as I remember them. Of course, they were in their seventies by then, so maybe they were at one time wildly sexual and just outgrew it by the time I met them. Most likely, the large families were the result of a lack of contraceptive knowledge and no TV to pass time in the evenings.

In any event, my mother was a single, divorced, working woman with a little daughter when my parents met, fell in love, and decided to get married. The year was 1932 - during the Great Depression. According to what my mother told me in later years, she became pregnant prior to the marriage. In those days, it was considered a very shameful situation. According to my mother, as much as they loved the large families they grew up in, my mother and father had definitely decided to have only two children. They made the choice to terminate the pregnancy for economic and social reasons, and their reasons were so compelling to them personally, that they chose an illegal abortion. Three years later, they had the additional child they planned on - ME. And, sticking to their original plan, they had no more children after me.

When I look back on this time in my family life, I don't see my parents as evil, baby-killing monsters. I see two people who were honest, hard-working, church-going Christians. They were two people who had lived in tough economic times, had plans for their life together, and who believed that life started at birth, not at the moment an egg was fertilized. They believed the choice they made was best for them and their choice to make. Perhaps this decision was made easier by the social and economic conditions, and it was apparently not too hard to do, even though it was illegal. My mother did not elaborate on the details. She merely told me that she had gone to a doctor and had it done. I guess that there were no organized protests about the procedure in 1932 and it had not become the all-consuming religious and political issue that it is today. One can call me selfish, but I am glad my mother had an abortion, legal or not, in 1932. Without it, I would not have been here, and I am a pretty important person - at least to me and to those who love me.

It has been said that we are a pill-popping culture. It's true that we consume a goodly number of the little devils.

We take pills to heal disease, control disease, and to prevent disease. We bolster our intake of valuable vitamins with pills. We lower our blood pressure and cholesterol with pills. We vanquish our aches and pains with pills. Everybody seems to take some pills and those precious pills are made available to everyone, young and old, healthy and sick, in an over-the-counter form or as a prescription from your doctor. There is no double standard when it comes to the availability of our precious pills, or is there? There is a double standard, or gender bias, when it comes to pills having to do with sex. The birth-control pill just celebrated its 50th birthday, theoretically being available for use for all of those fifty years. It was the first major breakthrough in contraception for women. However, the availability of the pill varied from state to state in the early days.

Paul:
When we lived in Massachusetts in 1958, the year we married, there were three options available for birth control: abstinence or the Catholic System of using timing, or "rhythm", which was not very successful and not suited to us newly-weds at the time, condoms, which were not completely safe and were also advertised "for the prevention of sexually transmitted disease only", and the diaphragm which, with spermicidal jelly, provided the best available protection

against unwanted pregnancy. We chose the latter, but, when the diaphragm, which was prescribed by a doctor in Illinois, got a hole in it, we could not get another in Massachusetts as it was against their law. We had to travel to another state to get the prescription refilled. This gender-based archaic law of Massachusetts prohibited a woman from obtaining a diaphragm, but did not prevent a man from obtaining a gross of condoms "for the prevention of sexually transmitted disease only".

Thanks to modern science, there are far more "magical" pills available when it comes to sexual function. Besides the "birth control" pill, there is now a pill known as "plan B", also known as "the morning after pill", RU486, and a plethora of erectile dysfunction drugs

The first major family planning breakthrough in the early 1960's, the birth control pill, has made contraception an easier issue. Although the birth control pill was approved by the FDA in 1960, its availability to women was not assured simply because of that approval. The birth control pill was not originally available in all states. It was not available until 1965 for married women (Griswold v. Connecticut), and not until 1972 for unmarried women (Eisenstaedt v. Baird). Talk about a double standard. In its early days, the birth control pill was roundly condemned by Right-to-Lifers. This was prior to the 1973 Roe v. Wade decision and, incidentally, prior to the modern "Pro-Life" movement. States opponents of the birth control pill argued that the birth control pill would increase sexual activity between unmarried couples and reduce the number of pregnancies. Both of these arguments were, perhaps, correct. The birth control pill may have encouraged a more active sex life by those without moral or religious compunction regarding pre-marital sex. It would also have reduced the number of unplanned or unwanted pregnancies affecting married and unmarried women. In both cases, so what? If I have moral or religious reservations regarding two consenting adults having a sexual relationship purely for pleasure and not procreation, should I be allowed individually or through my government, to prevent their action or make it more distressing for them by increasing the woman's chance of an unwanted pregnancy? Fortunately, the Supreme Court decided that contraception through the use of the birth control pill was in the realm of a woman's right to privacy in connection with her sexual conduct and her reproductive plans. In effect, it divorced sexual activity from reproduction by giving women control over their fertility. Looking at the big picture, it greatly affected our society by freeing women and allowing them to increase their numbers in our workforce.

The next sexual pill to appear on the scene was RU486. RU486 is a steroid compound called mifepristone. It is an abortifacient and in smaller doses acts as an emergency contraceptive. It was developed in France and first licensed there in 1988. Bowing to Pro-Life / Anti-Choice groups, the U.S. banned its use and availability in 1989. It was finally approved for abortion use in the U.S. in 2000 and is widely available.

However, the public cannot purchase it through pharmacies. It is only available through specially licensed physicians. Pro-Life /Anti-Choice and certain religious groups in the U.S. are quite naturally opposed to the legality of RU486 because they are opposed to abortion - period. They claim to address their objections from an "ethical" point of view. Pro-Choice groups naturally favor access to RU486 because they feel a woman's right to privacy, as far as her body is concerned, includes access to abortifacients.

Plan B (the morning-after pill) is an emergency contraceptive pill (ECP). ECP's contain higher doses of the same ingredient found in regular birth control pills. It was approved for use in the U.S. in the late 1990's. Morning after pills should not be confused with mifepristone, which acts as an abortifacient. They are contraceptives because they act prior to implantation/pregnancy. There is a medical and legal agreement on this issue. Because of this, ECP's are not considered effective in cases where a woman is already pregnant. As with other birth control issues in the past, the Anti-Choice movement geared up to make it difficult for women to use Plan B. It was originally available by prescription only and some pharmacies made it tough on a woman trying to get it. In 2003, an FDA advisory committee voted 23 to 4 to allow Plan B to be sold to women without a prescription, but a religiously conservative administration, catering to its political base, overrode these scientific advisors and squelched the recommended availability. This was partially reversed later, so that now, adult women may obtain Plan B without a prescription, but a girl under 18 may not. The battle rages on. Is Plan B an abortifacient? Technically, no. Does Plan B present a health hazard when it comes to other conditions like breast cancer, bowel disease, etc.? Studies show that there are no adverse effects. Does the availability of Plan B increase unprotected and irresponsible sexual behavior? Studies seem to show that contention is unfounded. Plan B is generally used as a backup in an emergency when a condom is torn or someone forgets to take a birth control pill. The idea that Plan B contributes to promiscuity is analogous to saying that having an emergency brake in a car contributes to making a person a bad driver.

The very latest pill being reviewed by the FDA, ulipristal acetate, is a new and improved ECP. It is already approved in forty-three countries and is known as Ella One. It has been found to be consistently effective up to 120 hours, or five days, after unprotected sex and may be twice as effective as Plan B. Anti-abortion activists want ulipristal acetate to be banned as an abortifacient, although it works by preventing the implantation of an egg.

Last in our review of precious pills, we need to mention the highly advertised erectile dysfunction pills. They do not need to be explained because they are advertised almost non-stop in nauseating detail on television. Although they are a prescription-only product, they flaunt an appeal to male sexual behavior without any apparent thought regarding the appropriateness of such advertising on our TV screens all day and night. How do you answer your 8 year old daughter when she asks, "Mom (or Dad), what is a 4 hour erection"? We have no doubt that a tasteful Plan B ad on television would be met with an uproar of conservative, religious indignation. Where is the uproar regarding these erectile dysfunction ads? Again, more gender-biased double standard!

DEFINITION OF HUMAN LIFE OR PERSONHOOD

The pro and con arguments regarding abortion and contraception all depend on the definition of human life. When does human life begin? In the Roe v. Wade decision, the Supreme Court justices concluded in Section IX that they did not feel they could make that determination since doctors, philosophers, and theologians were unable to arrive at a consensus. Our individual and corporate beliefs regarding human life vary greatly, from the moment the sperm penetrates the egg, to implantation (pregnancy), first heartbeat, viability (ability to survive outside the womb), ensoulment (whenever that is), to birth. Other ideas about when human life begins are determined by specific fetal development aspects, such as: 1st cell splitting, visible external body parts, brain waves, loss of gill slits, facial development, and all early developmental fetal characteristics, to later stages, such as the Jewish belief, when it is half-way emerged from its mother, all the way to a baby's breathing on its own. If a perfect full term baby arrives into this world and never takes a breath, there still is a question. Was it ever a living human person? There are many Bible passages which support breathing as a determinant of human life. Genesis 2:7 KJV says, "And the Lord God formed man of the dust of the ground, and breathed into his nostrils the breath of life: and man became a living soul". Also, in Genesis 6:17, God talks about destroying the earth by flood, "To destroy all flesh wherein is the breath of life" Most of the biblical argument used by "conceptionists" hinges on a song by David in Psalms 139:13, "For thou didst form my inward parts; thou didst weave me in my mothers womb". Aristotle believed that a male developed a soul some 40 days after conception, but it took some 90 days for a female fetus to develop her soul. More gender-based beliefs with no substantiation.

Today there are basically three "camps" of stance on abortion. In the Far Left Camp stands China, which because of its government policies regarding population, feels that it must have the right to mandate abortion against a woman's desires. The Far Right camp believes that the government should require every woman to carry to term every pregnancy, with no choice on her part, except in some circumstances, perhaps in cases of rape or threat to the mother's life. The Middle Camp desires to separate personal issues of morality and choice from governmental laws and mandates. If one's opinion on when human life begins places it at conception, that opinion then creates the problem of there then being two human beings involved in a decision regarding abortion choice, both having rights. As a member of the Middle Camp, it seems to me that a woman's right to control her body would certainly not be less than the rights of a yet-to-be fully-developed fetus. Should a fetus have the legal right to force a woman to undergo all of the physical and mental agonies of going through an unwanted pregnancy? The fetus, alone, does not have a choice - a woman does and should. Those who believe that a woman should only have the right to an abortion in the case of rape are the same people who believe that the fetus has rights from conception. Does the fetus caused by rape have fewer rights than the one which was planned and wanted? That position makes absolutely no sense to most logical-thinking people. The physical and mental trauma to a woman from having to undergo nine months of pregnancy and childbirth may be equally as great to her, whether it was caused by pleasurable sex or rape. The potentially human fetal tissue should have no right to demand control over a woman's body, if that is not her choice. The argument to retain the right to a safe abortion is supported by the figures regarding death rates of mothers when it was illegal to those when it became legal. Reducing abortion rates would certainly be a worthy goal from any viewpoint, especially from a cost factor, but rates should be reduced through educational measures and contraceptives. Personal risks of death from abortion and using contraceptives are far fewer than from carrying a pregnancy to term. Overturning Roe v. Wade would again cause an increase in maternal deaths. In other problem areas, such as drug use, alcohol abuse, and tobacco addiction, outlawing the abusive substance fills our jails, but does not have the effect for change and reducing abuse which education does.

It is very unfortunate that the Right Camp, stuck with their "conceptionist" mentality, leaves no room for compromise and abortion at any point in a pregnancy, or even prior to pregnancy (at conception). It is viewed as a heinous crime. The death threats, burning of abortion clinics, and killing of doctors who perform abortions are believed justifiable in their eyes because they prevent "killing babies". Dr. George Tiller, an abortion provider in Wichita, Kansas, was shot and killed in his church. He was described by a patient as an incredible, principled, and compassionate man, whose clinic was the only one in the U.S. providing late-term abortions. Only some 600 U.S. abortions a year, no matter the procedure, occur after the sixth month - all involving a tragically deformed fetus or a mother's life in peril. This patient was carrying her second child which would not survive birth. As she and her husband could not bear going through waiting for another loss, they went to Dr. Tiller. She told of his calling her some time after her procedure to ask her if she and her husband would like to adopt a baby which he had refused to abort.

After Dr. Tiller's death, a friend and medical colleague for over thirty years, Dr. Warren M. Hern, said in an address in Denver, "This is not just the personal tragedy of one abortion doctor, one honorable physician who took over his late father's family practice. This brutal, cold-blooded, premeditated political assassination is the inevitable and predictable result of over thirty-five years of rabid anti-abortion harassment, hate rhetoric, violence, and intimidation".

"CONCEPTIONIST"
CONCEPTIONS

"Conceptionists" beliefs raise many questions. About 50% of the fertilized ova develop into a baby. Some just never implant or become a pregnancy and some, fortunately, are miscarried because of abnormalities. Do "conceptionists" have funerals for every miscarriage? Should women be forced to spend half of their lives resting in bed to give the possibly-fertilized egg a good chance to implant? Pharmacists who are "conceptionists" are refusing to fill prescriptions for Plan B, RU486 and even the birth control pill.

Catholic dogma holds to the position that using any contraceptives is a sin. The sexual act is strictly relegated to marriage and, then, the intent should be strictly for procreation. Since Italy, the home of the Vatican, has one of the lowest birth rates of any country, it is obvious that Catholics there are pretty much ignoring the Pope and the church's bans. This is also true in other predominantly Catholic countries in Europe. In other sexual areas, the Catholic church has, shamefully, been in the forefront news-wise regarding their pedophile priests and their questionable handling of this sinful, illegal behavior. It is unbelievable to us, as non-Catholics, that a Catholic woman would have to confess her sin of using contraception to a priest who may be guilty of an immoral and illegal act against a child - who could be hers. Another Catholic dogma which most non-Catholics can not understand is that of requiring a doctor, faced with the decision between saving the life of the mother or child, to save the life of the child. How many dutiful Catholic mothers, unwillingly, leave this earth dumping a new-born and several other children on their disconsolate husbands? The logic escapes most pragmatic people.

In-vitro fertilization poses another dilemma for "conceptionists". In their zeal to have a baby, many of them can rationalize the use of fertility clinics, in-vitro fertilization, and the implantation of the resulting embryos into the womb. The fertility clinics extract a dozen or more eggs, fertilize them in dishes and then implant two or three in hopes that one or two will "take" and result in a child or two. The moral dilemma for the "conceptionist" is what to do with the extra fertilized eggs. If they are human beings, is it morally correct to freeze them for an undetermined period until they, perhaps, will also be able to be implanted and fulfill their destiny? Most are unneeded and destroyed because "conceptionists" believe that using them in research is wrong, although the cures for many diseases and genetic disorders may lie in their use. How do "conceptionists" rationalize the "death" of all the "babies" who aren't implanted or are destroyed because of their not being needed? A ludicrous, and in our thinking, immoral use of in-vitro fertilization occurred not too long ago when a fertility doctor implanted eight eggs into the womb of an unmarried woman who already had six children, resulting in eight more babies. Was it her right, alone, to chose to have fourteen children, depending on charity and the government to pay for their care? It was probably her legal right, but not a moral choice, but that's how we see it. What were the moral implications regarding the doctor's choice? Was his/her motive guided by anything other than monetary gain and notoriety?

Another problem "conceptionists" have is their lack of choice, because of their moral and religious beliefs regarding human life, when it comes to carrying all fetuses to term, if possible. A genetically imperfect fetus or grotesquely deformed fetus must be kept at all cost. The cost to the family, the child, and/or society may not be considered. From the persuasion of the Pro-Choice /"Middle Camp", it is allowable to consider all aspects of such a choice. What will be the effect on the parents and other children? What will be the financial costs of caring for a special-needs child? Will there be joys equal to the sorrows for the family of a special-needs child? What kind of life and what pain is the child going to endure? Most Pro-Choice people feel that parents and society have a moral obligation to care for a child after it is born no matter the cost, but modern medicine has thrown a hooker into that equation: Many severely damaged babies would die naturally if not treated at great cost with life-prolonging medical procedures. Is it moral to prolong the life of a baby for a minimal time at great medical cost when the outcome will be death anyway? Are the choices to treat at any cost moral? God knows - we don't - we guess. Some would call the choice to withhold out-of-the-ordinary treatment and allow natural death "infanticide". Infanticide, though most often considered wrong by all three "camps", actually only refers to the deliberate killing of a child, which unfortunately happens far too often when a baby becomes an inconvenience. Abortion is not infanticide, killing an already born baby is.

Per Wikipedia, the history of infanticide, now illegal in most of the world, although still practiced, is interesting. In many societies throughout time, certain forms of infanticide were actually allowed. Female killing has always been more prevalent than male because of the perceived desirability of males needed to do heavy work and go to war. Usually, natural selection produces 105-108 males per 100 females. Throughout known history, child sacrifice was practiced and infanticide was practiced at all times. It was practiced by all peoples, regardless of educational levels. Sacrifice of newborns was prevalent with evidence being found in Sardinia, Syria, and Egypt. Pelagians offered a sacrifice of every 10th child, (i.e., "to decimate" the populations) and Carthaginians, Phoenicians, Canaanites, Moabites and Sephardites offered their first-born as a sacrifice to their gods. Although practiced in Egypt at a later time, in ancient times taboos were in place forbidding infanticide. Greeks considered sacrifice to be barbarous, however, exposure of newborns was widely practiced. The exposed child had a theoretical chance of being rescued. A letter from a Roman citizen to his wife in 1 B.C. told her to let their child live if it was male, but to expose it, if it was female. Judaism prohibits infanticide, although there are several instances in the Bible of ancient Hebrews sacrificing their children to heathen gods. Josephus, a first century Jewish historian, wrote that God, "Forbids women to cause abortion of what is begotten, or destroy it afterward", however, 600 years earlier Jeremiah talked about the burning of infants as sacrifices to the god Molech. Early European tribes would kill a child before it had been given any food, especially in cases of out-of-wedlock children. There is evidence of burnt bones from child sacrifice in pagan Britain.

Christians rejected infanticide from the teachings of the Apostles onward. In 318 A.D. Constantine I decreed that all children should be raised, although exposing babies, especially females, was still common at the time. Although theologians preached saving all children, during the Middle Ages infanticide was practiced openly and on a large scale, with Romans throwing their newborns into the Tiber River during daylight. During that time, German mothers had the right to expose their newborns. When pagan Icelanders adopted Christianity, there were two concessions: Infant exposure was allowed, along with the eating of horse meat. Infanticide was practiced during pre-Islamic times, but explicitly prohibited by the Qur'an. In current times Muslims, although they may not practice infanticide, use the practice of honor-killings upon women who disgrace their family.

Even today infanticide is being practiced. Starting in 1986, women in New Guinea were killing their newborn male babies so their stock of males would go down and there would be no men in the future to fight - a very different, interesting way of stopping wars, but it probably won't be adopted widely outside of New Guinea. The United States ranks 11th in nations for killings of infants under one year of age. In the U.S. in 1983 over 600 children were killed by their parents. Today the reason for this practice is patrilineal, with sons more apt to support their parents until they die, and economic, with a family having more children than they can support, or to keep a stable population in line with resources. Postpartum depression is also related to infanticide and probably the cause of Andrea Yates drowning her five children, including a newborn.

Another related issue, infant euthanasia, occurs today around the world in cases where a newborn is severely impaired. Of the 200,000 children born each year in the Netherlands, 1,000 die during the first year of life. Of these 1,000, 600 are euthanized after a medical/parental decision. Many doctors believe it is right not to initiate and to withdraw life-prolonging treatment in newborns with no chance of survival and, because this practice is so common throughout the world, feel that it should be regulated. A Dutch protocol group separates severely ill newborns into three categories: those with no chance of survival, who will die soon regardless of medical care; those with a very poor prognosis and poor quality of life dependant on intensive care, and; those who experience what parents and experts feel is unbearable suffering. The Pro-Choice thoughts above differ from the Pro-Life in that the Pro-Life people believe that we must treat and care for all babies in as much as we are able. They base their arguments on the fact that severely medically affected children have survived infancy and are happy to be alive in spite of the suffering they have endured.

"Conceptionists" have started anti-abortion pregnancy centers all over the U.S.. These anti-abortion pregnancy centers go by some of the following names: Crisis Pregnancy Center, Pregnancy Aid, Open Door, Care Net, Birth Right Life Choices, or Pregnancy Counseling. Many such centers list themselves under "Abortion Services" in the advertising pages of the phone book. These are all run by Anti-Choice groups and a girl or woman who goes there would not have any choice or counseling regarding the option of not having to go through the pregnancy they are facing. In looking up seven Pregnancy sites on the internet in the Sylva, N.C. area, one turned out to be a spa for pregnant women, one was a Planned Parenthood site offering full services regarding sexual matters for men and women, and the other five were Pro-Life/Anti-Choice only, with such services as pregnancy tests, ultrasounds, and abortion recovery support groups. The real goal of these centers is to make women feel too guilty or scared to choose abortion through questionable counseling and inaccurate information.

NARAL Pro Choice America has identified 112 anti-abortion organizations who advertise in Yellow Pages.Com and Super Pages.Com under the heading "Abortion Services", although the directories have a category called, "Abortion Alternatives". These listings are clearly "purposefully deceptive", "false, misleading", and "fraudulent". In a U.S. House of Representatives minority report Henry Waxman concluded that CPC's provide false information regarding an alleged link between abortion and breast cancer, abortion and future fertility, and abortion and poor mental health. As of September 2006, there were over 2,200 CPC's in the U.S., most funded by one of the three major pro-life Evangelical and Roman Catholic organizations - Care Net, Heartbeat International, and Birthright International. In at least eight states, taxpayer money goes to subsidize Pro-Life CPC's and in seventeen states motorists can pay extra for "Choose Life" license plates. There has been no connection found between poor mental health and abortion, although pre-existing psychiatric illness, lack of support, and conservative anti-abortion counseling might increase negative feelings after an abortion. The American Psychological Association found that "severe negative reactions after an abortion are rare, but increase with multiple abortions, as well as with multiple unwanted pregnancies". The existence of what CPC's refer to as "post-abortion syndrome" is not recognized by any medical or psychological organization. It doesn't exist - the CPC's made it up. If faced with an unwanted pregnancy, a woman should first consider contacting Planned Parenthood. Their promise is: Creating hope for humanity, the freedom to dream, to make choices, and to live in peace with our planet. Choice would exist.

END OF
LIFE CHOICES

Barbara:
As a child of grammar school age, I vividly remember the death of my friend's father from bone cancer. Actually it was the dying process which haunts my memory. The death was a blessed event. The dying process went on for months and the neighborhood heard his screams of pain. From then on, I hated the fact that we could not help our loved ones escape their suffering like we could that of our animals. I remember "Punch" our beautiful black Cocker Spaniel puppy who ate some rat poison a neighbor had put out. The poison blinded him and made him very sick. Our family, together, decided that it was not "fair" to make our young puppy face a life of sickness and blindness. It was a choice we were able to make and since he couldn't talk to us and tell us what he wanted, I hope that we made the right decision. I felt that we did at that time and I have not changed my mind.

My uncle went for x-ray treatments for stomach cancer, which then spread to his brain and perhaps other places. I watched as my handsome uncle suffered for what seemed forever, and was reduced to a skeleton-like personage hardly resembling himself. What a sad time for his wife and young children, but heaven forbid, we should offer him an "early out"!

Hospice is an organization which helps with end of life care. It offers a form of palliative care rather than curative care. It is intended for patients with an end of life illness and provides a variety of services. Someone with a terminal illness will usually be eligible for hospice care if their doctor feels that, if the disease runs its normal course, there is a life expectancy of six months or less. One may also choose hospice care over other curative treatments for an illness. One need not have a specific terminal illness such as cancer, congestive heart failure, etc., to enter the Hospice program.

At age 104, my mother received Hospice care even though she had no specific disease. In her case, she was just wearing down - a "failure to thrive", as her doctor and Hospice put it.

Hospice is a great organization. Normally, it assists in providing care in the home, an assisted living facility, or a Hospice run facility. We have visited friends near death in a Hospice facility and found a loving, pleasant environment. Hospice coordinates care with the patient's doctors, but is at the patient's bedside frequently on a daily basis, which a doctor's schedule often will not allow. Hospice provides nurses, social workers, nurses aides, chaplain services, if desired, and medications for pain or anxiety relief. Hospice can also help in grief support and guidance in handling post-death arrangements. Most Hospice nurses are angels. They regularly visit patients in their care setting, usually in their home. They continually review the patients physical status, consult with their doctors, and monitor pain and anxiety medication dosages and consumption. They assist the caregiver (frequently a family member) in learning about medications and caregiver issues. Most people eligible for hospice care are over 65. Hospice is covered under Medicare. Frequently, other medical providers will pay for hospice care, but someone under 65 without health insurance would need to pay for hospice care. Some forms of financial assistance may be available for those with limited funds.

There are, however, instances in which Hospice care is not the answer. Hospice care can alleviate physical pain and suffering for terminal patients, but all patients are not terminal in six months, and all pain and suffering is not physical. A few years ago, our family went Christmas caroling at an assisted living facility. A very large percent of the residents were on public assistance. I will never forget one of the residents. She was in her mid-twenties and a few years earlier had been shot by her boyfriend during an argument. As a result of the gun shot wound, she was deaf, blind, and paralyzed. Perhaps she was kept free from physical pain, but can you imagine how she suffered? She was condemned to perhaps 40 more years of being unable to see, hear, or move from her bed.

Paul:

For a year before her death at 104, my mother needed to be dressed and undressed and helped to the dining room where she did not feel like eating much food. She could not go to the bathroom on her own, much less bathe or take a shower by herself. Perhaps, there are some people who would revel in this much attention, but, for my active, independent, creative mother, this was suffering.

Former Washington state governor, Booth Gardner, was diagnosed with Parkinson's disease. Gardner's disease, while debilitating, is not considered fatal by itself. Although Gardner realized that, after deteriorating health due to Parkinson's, death is the next step, there was little he could do to legally control his time of death. That, to an accomplished and active man, is a form of suffering.

Sir Edward Downes and his wife Joan were both celebrated artistic successes when Joan was diagnosed with incurable breast cancer. With Joan's terminal breast cancer, she faced a future of struggling to control pain and an ugly death. Sir Edward, who at 85 was becoming frail and losing his hearing and sight, faced an uncertain dim future of physical impairment without his beloved life's companion of 54 years.

What could these examples of suffering people do to alleviate their situations? In the case of the poor, blind, deaf, and paralyzed woman we encountered while singing carols at the assisted living facility, there is nothing she can do for herself. Any plea she might make to hasten her death would be ignored. She can only lie there in silent darkness and wait for death. What a maddening existence.

In the case of my 104 year old mother, if a magic pill to escape her debilitation had been available to her, I am sure that she would have seriously considered taking it. Although she had no specific terminal disease, she was just wasting away. To her, to be so frail that she even needed someone to wipe her bottom, was a real form of suffering. Although she was at most times alert and cheerful, at other times she was very anxious and fearful and she sat in her room crying, "Oh Lord, Lord, help me - why am I still here"?

Unfortunately, there was nothing she could do, nor could we help her end her suffering.

Booth Gardner decided that he would try to help others escape the loss of control over the end of their lives. He spearheaded an effort to pass a law in Washington similar to Oregon's Death With Dignity Act. The Death With Dignity Act allows patients who have less than six months to live, certified by two physicians, to obtain prescriptions from their doctors for enough drugs to kill themselves. There are enough legal safeguards to protect against abuse or the killing of someone without their consent. Ten years of experience in Oregon clearly showed that the Death With Dignity Act was not frequently used (from 1998 through 2006, only 292 people actually died by using this process) and it had not turned into the "slippery slope" towards involuntary euthanasia claimed by the act's opponents. Nevertheless, the Washington measure, like the Oregon action which preceded it, was vigorously opposed by the Roman Catholic Church and various Right-To-Life groups. The members of the Washington State Medical Association were split on the issue. In spite of the well-financed campaign against it, in 2008, the measure passed and Washington became the second state to allow for physician assisted suicide for terminally ill patients. Since then, Montana became the third state to allow this procedure when its courts ruled that the right to privacy extends to terminal patients seeking a doctor's help in ending their lives. Perhaps, Booth Gardner's crusade was his way of handling the situation he faced.

What about the Downeses? Joan Downes decided that she did not want to experience the pain and suffering which would be caused by her terminal illness. Sir Edward Downes, faced with unavoidable physical decline and the certainty of an impaired and feeble old age, decided that he would rather not continue to live without Joan. The Downeses went to a clinic in Switzerland. Assisted suicide is legal in Switzerland. There, the Downeses took lethal doses of a drug, quickly falling unconscious, and dying peacefully, holding hands.

We believe that people should be allowed to make their own end of life decisions. One argument against allowing assisted suicide is that God, not humans, should determine the time we die. That argument overlooks the fact that God has apparently been delegating death for years. From the violent tales of conflict and death in the Bible's Old Testament, to the Crusades, to the Inquisition, to history's many wars, just and unjust, to our forefathers policy of Manifest Destiny, to modern extremists killing in the name of God, death has been meted out by one human group upon another. In most of those cases, the recipients of the death have not been suffering or asking for release from this world. The argument that the time of death is entirely God's decision does not seem to hold water.

Another argument against allowing assisted suicide is that it will lead down a "slippery slope" to the murder of old people for financial gain. Assisted suicide is legal in the Netherlands, Belgium, and Switzerland, as well as in three states in the U.S.. Legal safeguards in all of these locations have proved that the "slippery slope" is rhetorical and does not exist.

Still another argument made against legalizing assisted suicide is that once we declare assisted suicide a legal right, people suffering from non-terminal conditions such as spinal cord injuries, debilitating handicaps, and non-terminal depression and despair, might opt for that choice. How many people are there in those categories who are suffering and would like to choose the time of their death? I don't know what they, or the woman in the assisted living facility, would decide. But, I do believe that the decision regarding if or when to end their existence should be theirs to make.

There are many people in our society who are suffering. Their physical pain can often be alleviated, but in some cases pain killing drugs are withheld or rationed to the point that the suffering from pain continues. Some of these people are terminal within six months. Others are not. There are many patients who suffer from progressively incapacitating diseases such as emphysema, Lou Gehrig's disease, cancer, advanced cases of Parkinson's, etc. There are people who have been diagnosed with early stages of Alzheimer's disease who dread the thought of progressing down a narrowing tunnel of dementia to a vegetative state for several years, causing an emotional drain and financial burden for their families and loved ones. Until recently, their only escape was a frequently messy, sometimes painful, and not always successful attempt at suicide, or a trip to Switzerland.

Now, the right to assisted death exists in a very limited and controlled way, in the states of Oregon, Washington, and Montana. One more alternative opened up in 2004 with the formation of Final Exit Network. Final Exit Network is not a "suicide club". It is a non-profit 501(c) (3) educational association which tries to help people who feel their lives are so miserable that they no longer want to live. Final Exit Network's guiding principle is, "Mentally competent adults have a basic right to end their lives when they suffer from a fatal or irreversible illness or intractable pain, when their quality of life is personally unacceptable, and the future holds only hopelessness and misery. Such a right shall be an individual choice, including the timing and companion, free of any restrictions by law, clergy, medical profession, even friends and relatives no matter how well-intentioned. We do not encourage anyone to end their life, do not provide the means to do so, and do not actively assist in a person's death. We do, however, support them when medical circumstances warrant their decision". Final Exit Network recommends and explains the use of helium as a very effective method of ending life. It is rapid, gentle, and pain-free. Although Final Exit Network does not require that one's affliction needs to be terminal within a short time, it does require that one be mentally competent before it will provide its educational guidance regarding the end of life process. Exit guides are trained and caring persons and often have several meetings with the person asking for deliverance before making the decision to counsel that person on how to "self-deliver". Guides may or may not be with the person at the time of death, but do not assist in their death. It is interesting to note that no states have laws against a person committing suicide, but all states have laws against assisting in a suicide. It seems odd to have a law against helping a person do something which is legal, but that's the way it is. Final Exit Network, through its right to free speech, provides detailed educational information on its recommended method of hastened death, but does not physically assist in hastened death in any way. Final Exit Network has been harassed by legal authorities in Georgia, who were no doubt spurred on by the "Right Camp" contingency.

Assisted suicide has been fought by several influential groups. The Catholic Church and Right-to-Life groups oppose it because of religious beliefs. Some physicians oppose it for various reasons. They may feel that their overriding duty is to be a force for life, not death. Even though they might want to help, some may fear legal prosecution, and let's face it, some doctors, hospitals, and nursing homes benefit financially from the prolongation of life. Opposition to suicide or terminating life "early" can also come from friends or family who simply don't want to lose a loved one.

One of the most tragic and bizarre events in the end-of-life struggle was the Terri Schiavo affair. Terri Schiavo was a young Florida woman who was in a coma for years and was deemed brain-dead by her attending physicians. She was kept breathing by a ventilator and nourished by a feeding tube at great financial cost, first through private and later by public funding. Her inability to communicate or respond for years, along with a completely negative medical prognosis, resulted in her husband's decision to ask that she be detached from life-support. He claimed that Terri had always said that she would not want to be kept alive in this manner, although he could not prove that through a written document. Terri's parents objected to discontinuing artificial life support systems, perhaps a normal reaction from grieving parents. The matter went through the court system with Republican politicians, including Florida's Republican governor, and their Right-to-Life supporters vociferously opposing the intent of Mr. Schiavo. When the Florida Supreme Court ruled in Mr. Schiavo's favor and the Federal Courts declined to intervene, the congressional Republicans called a special session in the nation's capital to pass a bill ordering the Federal Courts to intervene in the matter. The religiously conservative, Right-to-Life president at the time, flew back to Washington D.C. from his vacation home in Texas, specifically to sign the legislation. Of course, the legislation was blatantly unconstitutional. We have a separation of powers in this country and the legislative branch cannot order the judicial branch to do whatever the legislative branch desires. The legislation, though passed, went nowhere. Finally, Mrs. Schiavo's artificial life support systems were disconnected and she died shortly after. A subsequent autopsy revealed that her brain had completely deteriorated and a return to a conscious life state was impossible. Besides proving the need for having one's end-of-life desires in written form, the Terri Schiavo case clearly illustrates the extent to which the Right-to-Life/Anti-Choice movement will go to pursue its goal of "life-above-all else" and the hold it has on one of our country's major political parties.

Whatever you may think about Jack Kervorkian aside, in a June, 2010 interview he said he wants to keep living because he has three missions. He wants to tell mankind about "impending doom". He worries that our culture of over-abundance will soon lead to the extinction of the human race. His second mission is to educate people about what he has termed "patholysis" which is bringing an end to suffering. He feels that the Oregon, Washington, and Montana laws are not adequate in that a person has to be considered terminal in order to qualify for assisted death. He asks, "What difference does it make if someone is terminal? We are all terminal". His third mission is to convince the American public that their rights are infringed upon every-day - and, he feels that the Ninth Amendment is not being upheld. He believes that the amendment calls for protection of the rights to assisted suicide, euthanasia, and "patholysis," as well as the right to smoke in public places.

The ninth amendment was put into the Bill of Rights because there was a fear on the part of the Anti-Federalists that in naming some liberties in the Bill of Rights, they would imperil others. The ninth amendment became the protector of unnamed liberties. It was not addressed until 1965 when it was used in the Supreme Court case Griswold

v. Connecticut regarding a Connecticut law which banned adult residents from using birth control. The majority opinion was based on the interpretation that fundamental personal rights should not be denied protection simply because they are not specifically listed in the Constitution. After Griswold, federal courts were flooded with unusual claims based on "unnamed rights", with most rejected, as, I am sure would also be, Kevorkian's "right to smoke in public places"

Not Dead Yet was founded on April 27, 1996, shortly after Jack Kervorkian was acquitted in the assisted suicides of two women with non-terminal disabilities. Since then, eleven other national disability rights groups have taken action in over thirty states and helped put Kervorkian in jail in 1999. In the 2003-2005 fight to save Terri Schiavo, twenty-five disability rights groups joined Not Dead Yet in opposing her guardian's right to "starve and dehydrate her to death". All of the disability rights groups reasons for existence are based on unsubstantiated "slippery slope" politics. All Right-to-Die groups reasons are based on a competent person's personal desires to choose when he/she dies and have NO effect on any person who does not choose to die.

Some would argue that allowing a person in a non-terminal condition the right to assisted suicide would cheapen life and be inhuman. However, how does the time one chooses to depart this life deal in any way with a perceived cheapening of that life? To the contrary, one would think that allowing a person to make such a decision would be a recognition that life is one's most precious possession. Should government, religious institutions, or medical societies have control of our most precious possession or should we have it? Who is the final arbiter of our suffering - others or we? All of the arguments for or against voluntary early termination of life can, in the final analysis, be set aside. No one has the right or obligation to extend the suffering of another person. In the end, it boils down to a matter of choice - our choice.

THEOCRACY VERSUS DEMOCRACY

Radical right Christians and radical Islamists, although naming each other as "holy enemies", favor each other in many beliefs. Each is totally intolerant of beliefs other than their own. They favor male domination over women and sexual repression and use violence to uphold their beliefs. In times of uncertainty and despair, it is easy to blame the "scapegoats" for the problems which exist and search for promise, hope, and validation through the Spiritual. They await release in the promise of apocalyptic books like the "Left Behind" series by La Haye and Jenkins. Those who are not "saved" will be responsible for all the suffering which comes to them. They become more clannish, inward-looking, and condemning, and have little compassion for those on welfare. Compassion and financial support are basically reserved for those who believe as they do. Because submission to God's will (God generally being a male figure) is an important factor in the "Right Camp" and men need the justification of the their maleness, women are expected to submit to them. In the "Right Camp" view there is a clear demarcation between right and wrong, or "their way" and "sin". They must bury unclean thoughts and deny bad motives and fears. They validate their certainty by creating their own brand of morality.

James Dobson, who founded "Focus in the Family" and the lobbying arm, "Family Research Council" is reported to be anti-choice, anti-gay, pro prayer-in-school, pro-creationism, anti stem-cell research, pro male dominance and female submission, pro-abstinence-only sex education, and pro-guns. He has promised never to back any political candidate who is not "Pro-Life". Dobson has said Roe v. Wade unleashed the biggest "Holocaust" in world history and has compared the black robes of the Supreme Court Justices to the white robes of the K.K.K.

The Radical Right has their own belief system based on opinion, rather than fact. Much actual fact is disregarded and dismissed by them as wrongful opinion. Facts are only utilized when they fit in with their belief system. They disseminate books and articles which try to legitimize and substantiate their erroneous beliefs. They challenge scientific research regarding evolution, contraceptives, and global warming. Their aim is to spread their beliefs by political means rather than simply being concerned about their own personal salvation and personal morality. They look at this as a war against immorality which must be won politically. They hold rallies in which all who don't agree with their belief system are denounced as "secular humanists", "secular environmentalists", liberals, and pagans. They make promises of personal and collective salvation from economic woes and a sinful world. Democracy is seen as an enemy of faith, in that it keeps religion private, separate, and is tolerant of all faiths. They, of the Christian Right, are intolerant of homosexuals, Pro-Choicers, evolutionists, those favoring gun control, environmentalists, and people who are concerned about global population and global warming. They call ecological catastrophes acts of God's displeasure and deny any human cause. To them, God alone, is responsible for all human fate. Jerry Falwell went so far as to say that the 9-11 terrorism was God's punishment for all the abortions performed in this country. The Radical Christian Right in this country calls for intolerance and cruel acts against those who do not fall in line with their beliefs and these actions are perpetrated in the name of God. The End justifies the Means. Blaise Pascal said, "Men never do evil so completely and cheerfully as when they do it from religious conviction". Some of the worst atrocities in human history have been perpetrated by those seeking only to enforce their narrow version of what is correct and good on others. Their idealism allows, no compels, them to change or suppress those who don't believe as they do. They must and do have the right in our Democracy to believe and worship as they choose, but they should not be allowed to create a Theocracy where they can limit the choices of other citizens according to their spiritual beliefs.

A case in point which tragically shows the Radical Right's intention to control a woman's right-to-choice politically, also stars Florida's Ex-Governor Jeb Bush, famous for his part in the Terri Schiavo debacle.

In May 2003, he asked the courts to appoint a guardian for the fetus of a 22 year old rape victim. This woman was in the care of the state's adult protective services, living in a group home and raped, allegedly by the owner's husband. She had cerebral palsy, was autistic, needed help in bathing and walking, and could not identify the rapist due to her mental and physical state. Although the Supreme Court had said that a fetus does not count as a person under the 14th amendment, Bush "believed", due to his religious convictions, and directly in opposition to existing law, that it was appropriate to intervene. The Department of Children and Families initially said it would seek a guardian for the woman's child after it was born, but Bush and Jerry Regier, the secretary of the agency, decided that the agency should make the request for the fetal guardianship. Bush and Regier are strong abortion opponents and, even though abortion was not an issue in this case, Anti-Choice groups are pushing for the legalization of "fetal rights" every time they see an opportunity. The needs of the severely handicapped woman were not taken into consideration, only the "rights" of the unborn fetus. " If a guardian is appointed (fetal) there would be a clear recognition that there is a human being occupying that womb" said Brian Fahling, senior trial lawyer for the American Family Association's Center for Law and Policy.

Tragically the woman's disability, which should have entitled her to special government care, instead was used to make a case for forcing religious morality upon all citizens, through changes in political law regarding "fetal rights." If a pregnant women's actions regarding her body can be dictated by the needs of her fetus, imagine the severe, draconian restrictions which could be imposed on every pregnant woman.

Perhaps some historical perspective would be useful. Although our founding fathers were mostly Christians, (some notable exceptions were Benjamin Franklin and

Thomas Jefferson, who were deists) the Declaration of Independence does not mention Christianity. It mentions God once. Of course, the Declaration of Independence is not the document that formed our government. Instead, it is a statement that thirteen colonies no longer owed their allegiance to a distant, foreign king. Eleven years after the Declaration of Independence, our Constitution was written. It is the document which formed our government. Our Constitution does not once mention Jesus Christ or God. As noted earlier in this book, it does, however, specify that our government will not establish a religion or have any religious requirement for office.

Furthermore, in 1797, John Adams, our second president, signed the Treaty of Tripoli. Noted historian, David Mc Cullough, has called John Adams possibly the most religious of all U.S. presidents. Adams was around for the signing of the Declaration of Independence and the Constitution. He served as George Washington's vice-president for eight years. The Treaty of Tripoli specifically states that the U.S. is not a Christian nation. It should be noted that, according to our Constitution, treaties once passed and signed become the law of the land. It is certainly clear that the U.S. was not founded as a theocracy.

The inherent problems which would be brought to the forefront by America's becoming a Theocracy would not be unlike those of today's Saudi Arabia government, whose Sharia law is based on the Qur'an, the Law of Allah. The children's schools study math, The Qur'an, Hadith, and memorize the ninety-nine names of Allah. By any civilized standard, this Islamic law is demeaning to women, barbaric in its justice system, and intolerant of other religious faiths. The same may be said of the current theocratic government in Iran, and to a lesser and varying degree in other countries under Islamic influence.

In 1920 in Egypt, the Islamist revivalist movement, The Muslim Brotherhood, started with the goal to establish the "Kingdom of God" on earth for everyone. Women had to cover completely and wear flat shoes and use no perfume. A man's sinful, erotic thoughts were blamed directly on women. A marriage neither required the signature of the woman involved nor her presence. These are typical restrictions of Sharia law.

According to Muslim scholar Fazlur Rahman, "Islam insisted on the assumption of political power since it regarded itself as a repository of the Will of God which had to be worked on earth through a political order…To deny this fact would be to violate history and to deny justice to Islam itself".

Nezir Hyseni has written that "Islam is a political, cultural, and religious system. Religion, as based primarily on the Qur'an is a "part" of the system. Religious doctrine, however, is viewed in Islam as a preamble to Islamic law, the Sharia (divine law), which is a comprehensive code governing every aspect of life, because Islam is a religion primarily oriented toward law rather than theology". We have found it difficult to get a clear picture of exactly what is said in the Qur'an because the translations vary to such a large degree and there is no official translation of the Qur'an in English. In fact, there is no translation in any language which is considered official. The only language in which the Qur'an is considered correct is Arabic, so to really get the correct meaning you would have to be fluent in Arabic. We found that Ayaan Hirsi Ali's book "Infidel" gave a clear inside view of life under Islamic laws and culture from a woman's perspective. As a child she was subjected to the gross torture of genital mutilation, beatings by men and women alike, and expected to accept as a husband anyone her father might choose, all because it was, "The Will of Allah". Her journey to escape the "mind-forged manacles" of theocracy is a fascinating read. She also says, "In the Muslim world there is hardly a self, because the only real human moments are stolen ones. This leads to hypocrisy, which is the main cause of self-righteousness". We feel that there are many moderate Muslims who wish to be peaceful and tolerant and it behooves them to work for a reformation in Islam to a faith which is more compatible with the modern world. It seems that in many places in our world the moderate Muslims are losing ground, rather than gaining it.

Paul:
In 1992, I gave a series of lectures at universities across the island of Java in Indonesia. My wife and I were accompanied by a driver and guide. Our guide was a lovely young woman named Ipung. Ipung had a master's degree in accounting from a U.S. university and was hoping to pursue

her education further and become the first Indonesian woman to earn a PhD in accounting. Ipung was also a devout Muslim. During our trip, I was informed that on one Thursday we would have an extra day off because it was a religious holiday. When I asked what religious holiday it was, Ipung laughed and told me it was a Christian holiday - Ascension Day. It was then I learned that, at that time, Indonesia recognized important holidays for all the major religions. On that day off, we stopped in a village to pay a visit to Ipung's "auntie" who turned out to be a Christian. It was obvious that Ipung and her aunt adored each other. There was no tension between the Muslim young woman and her Christian aunt. At that time, there were a few remote areas in Indonesia which non-Muslims were encouraged to avoid because of extremists but, in general, religious animosity seemed minimal and we were treated very cordially by friendly people.

Today persecution of non-Muslims has been spreading in Indonesia. Since 1996, 786 Christian churches have been burned, attacked or closed throughout Indonesia. Although Indonesia's national constitution guarantees religious freedom, several extremist Muslim groups are active and have even intimidated and threatened government officials, police and judges.

At the present, we do not seem to hear a strong voice from these moderates condemning Sharia law and extremist terrorism. Are they afraid to speak out, even in this country, for fear of retaliation?

The inhuman act of those 9-11 Muslim hijackers was the logical outcome of a detailed system for regulating human behavior. The radical Muslim world is divided between "Us and Them" - if you don't accept Islam, you should perish. They believe that there can be no government without Allah and his book of laws for the conduct of worldly affairs. This form of government, be it Muslim, Christian, Buddhist, Hindu, or other denies choice. What form of government do you want? Theocracy or Democracy - that is your choice.

CHOICE
IN JOBS

Choice in a free society has to include the ability to select a profession, trade, or economic endeavor, through which we can diligently apply ourselves in gainful employment so as to achieve a relatively comfortable life for ourselves and our loved ones. Not very long ago, a person without a university degree could find sufficient gainful employment in manufacturing, building trades, or upper level service industries. Those workers could live well, own their own homes, and educate their children in hopes that they would have a chance to live even better lives than their parents. In those days, a university degree opened many doors - but a high school education was adequate. Poor and lower middle class Americans had the realistic opportunity to move into the middle class. Is that important? I think it is. We should all want to reduce poverty and see our fellow Americans experiencing a decent lifestyle. We should also not forget that the middle class is the main contributor to a stable society, not only in the U.S., but elsewhere. Look around the world and you will see that countries without a large middle class tend to be unstable and backward politically, economically, and socially. In some of these backward countries, the richest

1% of the population takes in as much as 20% of the total income of the country. Shocking you might say, but we are now, as a country, facing worse statistics than those banana republics. The wealthiest 1% of Americans now earn almost 24% of our total income. In 1976, that same 1% earned 9% of the income. The difference has been lost by our shrinking middle class. CEO's of the largest American companies today earn 531 times as much as their average worker - up from 42 times in 1980.

Today, America has forty million under-educated people in her workforce. Advances in technology and specialization, along with increased educational opportunities, mean that in America's current modern economy everyone with a high school education or less (about 40 million of us) is under-educated. Unfortunately, job opportunities for those in our under-educated workforce have been drastically reduced in recent years. A loss of manufacturing jobs in the United States has dramatically changed our economic structure. While improved workplace efficiency has resulted in the loss of some jobs, NAFTA and the globalization of the world's economy have been the most serious causes of our loss of manufacturing jobs. Too often, we hear of companies closing factories in the U.S. and re-opening them across the border in Mexico, where wages are very low and benefits and environmental rules are practically non-existent. The manufactured goods are then sent back to the U.S. duty-free. That, of course, may be helpful for corporate profits because the company profit margin is higher due to its reduced manufacturing cost, and in many cases, the avoidance of U.S. corporate income tax.

Also, it can be beneficial to the American public, at least to those who still have their jobs, as some corporations may reduce the prices for their product. Canada is our largest source for oil (not Saudi Arabia as some might think) and we in America can import their oil and natural gas without any tariffs. That, too, is a benefit.

Because the U.S. did lose more jobs than it gained in various industries due to NAFTA, during the 2008 presidential campaign McCain, Clinton, and Obama all agreed that NAFTA was a mistake, even though Mexico and Canada have benefited job-wise from NAFTA. Of course, corporate outsourcing has not been entirely because of NAFTA. Our corporations have moved untold numbers of manufacturing jobs to far-flung countries, most notably, China. This has been the main cause of our country's precipitous drop in domestic manufacturing jobs.

Just how bad has our loss of manufacturing jobs been? Consider this. In 1965 manufacturing jobs made up 53% of our economy. In 1988, it was 39%. In 2004, it was down to 9%, which was the first time since our industrial revolution that less than 10% of America's workforce has been employed in manufacturing. Our 40 million under-educated American workers face another obstacle besides dwindling manufacturing jobs. That obstacle is the illegal immigrant worker. Official estimates indicate that we have about 12 million of them in the U.S., although some people estimate the number to be much higher. What we know about our illegal immigrant workers is that they are generally under-educated and represent the low end of the societies from which they come. They are willing to work hard and put in long hours for sub-standard wages. They endure living conditions which are beneath ideal American standards and many times they are sending much of their earnings back to the country of their origin to help alleviate the poverty there. The illegal immigrants have secured employment in many of our remaining factories. Notable examples are the carpeting and meat-packing facilities, as well as our building trades and service industries. A paper on immigration and jobs written by Donald L. Huddle in 1992 contained the following observation and prediction, "The growth of the working age population in Mexico, Central and South America in the next three decades will dwarf that of the United States..... there is no prospect that all of these people will find jobs at home. Many of them will seek to come to the United States, as a matter of survival, and the problems of competition with unskilled American and legal residents labor will intensify rather than fading away". It has happened.

Paul:
Let me give a few examples of the changes I have personally seen. One summer during my college years, I worked for a landscaping company. All of my fellow workers were Americans. My best friend worked construction during the summers. His co-workers were Americans. Any of my high school friends who did not go on to college worked in the building trades and up

until a few years ago, I always saw that the framers, plasterers, etc., in the construction crews were Americans. We have had roofs replaced on various properties during our 40 years in Florida. Up until the last one five years ago, the roofing crews were mostly American. Our last roofing crew was made up mostly of what appeared to be illegal Hispanic immigrant workers from Latin America. Why should that be an important concern for our country? After all, these illegal (undocumented) workers may be under-educated, but they are poor, need the money, and work hard for longer hours and less pay than our American workforce. The argument that our illegal workers are poor, come from countries without the opportunities offered in America, and work hard is true. But, that is true for most of the world. The world is full of poor people who work hard and would love to be here, but we can not take them all in. We already have 40 million under-educated American workers who need employment in our factories, trades and service industries. If we fill those jobs with illegal immigrants, what will we do with our own under-educated workers?

An argument is made that illegal workers only take the jobs that Americans will not do. To an extent, that is true in agriculture. However, most of our 1-3 million migrant agricultural workers are seasonal and about half of them have no legal status in the U.S. The other half are legal workers under our H-2A Agricultural Guest Worker Program. Many agricultural employers do not participate in the government's Agricultural Guest Worker Program because they want to pay their workers even less. It is true that present wages and living conditions in agriculture are generally so poor that most Americans would refuse the work. I, for one, would feel terrible about imposing those conditions on any fellow American. So, as a nation, our choice is to impose poverty level wages and horrible living conditions on agricultural migrant workers, both legal and illegal, or to increase the wages to a decent American standard so Americans will take these jobs . We may have to pay more for tomatoes.

Since no more than 15% of our undocumented immigrant workers are in agriculture, it is obvious that we have shifted from a migrant agricultural workforce to an illegal immigrant industrial workforce. Are these jobs which no American will take? Twenty-five years ago jobs in the meat-packing plants were among the highest paid industrial jobs in the nation. Now illegal immigrants have taken over those positions and the pay for those jobs has decreased. A frequently made pro-illegal immigrant argument is that the illegals take jobs Americans don't want. Not true! Studies have shown that Americans will take 80% of the jobs filled by illegals with agriculture being the possible exception. However, we have a migrant guest worker program which could handle that 15% of the twelve million illegals. Of course, American and legal immigrant workers who take those jobs would need to be paid a decent wage subject to income and payroll taxes. The labor cost to some employers would be higher, but the cost to society as a whole would be less. Americans will work in plants, factories, construction, and service industries if given wages which will allow them to maintain a decent standard of living. New illegal immigrants will always be willing to work for less money. The fact that they are here illegally, and dirt poor to boot, leaves them with no choice.

Employers benefit from illegal immigrant labor because it increases their profits, but one certainly may question whether that benefit makes up for the lack of employment opportunities for our 40 million under-educated workers who are already suffering from the reduction of available manufacturing jobs caused by NAFTA and other outsourcing. Unemployment can create stress in marriages, an increase in crime, despondence, and other social ills. Most illegal immigrant workers put additional strain on our medical services, since their jobs seldom include benefits of any kind and their economic level precludes them from purchasing any medical insurance. Public schools also feel the strain. When my cousin moved here, legally, from Germany thirty years ago, her eight year old son spoke no English. He was enrolled in a public school and had to learn English. There were no bi-lingual teachers for him. It was tough for him, but with his mother's help he learned quickly and soon fit in. Today, our schools spend an unnecessary amount of our scarce education dollars teaching classes in Spanish as well as English. This expenditure is wasteful and doesn't achieve the assimilation we have always desired for our immigrants, so that they can feel a part of our country.

Think of the extra costs to our government of their having to print license and other forms in Spanish. If an immigrant is legal, he/she should know enough English to read forms, or bring an interpreter with him/her. If a Spanish-speaking person is living in this country and working in this country and expects the benefits our country offers, the least he/she should do is to learn English and fast. I believe that the primary secondary language which should be taught in our schools is Spanish, as it is an important language which is spoken by millions of our neighbors. I find it very offensive to see all signage in our English speaking country becoming dual English/Spanish. I refuse to shop in a store I once frequented which has big signs on their walls, Dresses/Vestidos and Shoes/Zapatos.

At the present time, our country is facing tough economic times and many Americans are upset with what they see as an illegal immigrant problem. For economic and security reasons, they want the illegals to leave and our borders sealed to all but controlled legal immigration. They see our need for educated legal immigrants, who will not compete with our own forty million under-educated workers for scarce jobs. Illegal immigrant advocates argue that our government can not logistically or economically pay for sending the illegals back home. True, but if our government were to initiate stiff fines on employers of illegals, with the possibility of jail time for repeat offenders, the illegal job market would disappear and the undocumented workers would just go home - on their own. They found their way here without help from our government and they could surely find their way back home again without help, if no jobs were available.

The establishment of a system of employer fines will probably not occur. Instead, various organizations are advocating amnesty for our twelve million or so illegal worker immigrants. Generally, they do not call it amnesty. Instead, they substitute something like "A path to citizenship" and window-dress it with, "They must learn English", "They must pay back taxes", "They must pay a (very nominal) fine", "They must go to the end of the line", etc. "Hogwash", it boils down to amnesty. In 1986 when Reagan gave amnesty to three million illegals, it was to take care of the problem and the prevention of further illegals crossing our borders was to have been handled by border patrols and fencing. With twelve million additional illegals here now, you can see how effective that program has been. Amnesty advocates include the Democrat Party (they see more Democrat votes from an increase in eligible Latino voters), elements of the Republican Party (whose corporate benefactors see economic benefits from being able to hire from an increased under-educated worker pool), labor unions (who see an opportunity to increase their flagging union membership), and Latino groups (who see it as an ethnic and power issue).

The truth is that amnesty or the present illegal worker situation, combined with our huge loss of domestic manufacturing jobs, means disaster for the American blue collar wage earner. This, in turn, can spell deep societal problems for our country in the future. We have about forty million under-educated (by modern standards) Americans in our workforce. These people are here - now - and they are not going away. As a country, we need to bring back as much of our manufacturing base as we can and open our jobs to American workers. That means we might have to pay our gardeners $20.00 an hour rather than $10.00 or pay $20.00 for a new shirt, instead of $10.00. What alternative do we have? We can't place forty million under-educated American workers as greeters at Walmart.

SEX EDUCATION
AND CHOICE

All young people deserve to be educated early in life regarding factual sexual function. During the sexually repressive "Right Camp" years, sex education became solely "abstinence only" sex education. The teaching of the social, physiological, and health gains to be realized by abstaining from or postponing sexual activity should be a primary factor in a sex education program, but certainly not the only factor being taught, as has been the case for some years. To simply teach, "Just Say No", is naïve and destructive to our youth. There are many good arguments which certainly should be promoted regarding the positive reasons for abstinence as well as the many negative results from early sexual relationships. "Right Campers" have felt that it is best to teach young people that all they need to know about sex is that it should not be practiced until marriage, and if they do, they will be justifiably punished by unplanned pregnancy, STD's, and death. Real sex education has been replaced by "Right Camp" theology - ignorance and fear in preference to correct information.

Eric Keroack, chosen by Bush to head family planning programs at the Department of Health and Human Services had, as medical director of "A Woman's Concerns", a network of CPC's in Massachusetts, spread the myth that having an abortion increased the risk of breast cancer. He also stated that the distribution of contraceptive drugs and devices was degrading of human sexuality and adverse to human health and happiness. Another claim of his was that sex with multiple partners altered brain chemistry making it harder to form bonding relationships - complete pseudo-science.

We are suffering the consequences of this backward step in sex education by high numbers of sexual diseases and unwanted pregnancies. From 1996-2004, 700 million dollars of taxpayers money were wasted on "abstinence only" education and, in order to get federal funding for such programs, educators were only allowed to follow those guidelines. Planned Parenthood called "abstinence only" education, "An experiment gone awry", and claimed that the 1.5 billion spent on it brought forth not one positive aspect. Other figures show that from 73 million per year was spent in 2001 to 204 million in 2008. Yes, 1.5 billion in federal money (yours and mine) spent on an ideology. A Johns Hopkins study showed that between the teens who took the abstinence pledge and those who did not, there was no difference in their sexual behavior, or the age at which they began having sex, or the numbers of their partners. Sadly, young people who received "abstinence only" education were less likely to use condoms when they did have sex and have suffered the consequences.

Most parents (over 90%) support comprehensive sex education and want discussions to include abstinence, sexual orientation, abortion, STD's, and the psychological aspects of sexual activity. Many health groups and religious groups, along with 8 in 10 conservative Christians, support comprehensive sex education. Why has a vocal minority been allowed to pressure schools and politicians into forcing such a lame excuse for sex education on our young for so long? Thank heavens, our 2008 elections brought in some politicians interested in promulgating comprehensive sex education. Using specially trained comprehensive sex education teachers is probably preferable to forcing the teaching of a touchy subject on unwilling, uncomfortable, and possibly unqualified teachers. From the personal experience we had as young people and then as parents regarding sex education, we wish that there had been such experts available during those past times. Students need help from trained counselors and teachers in understanding their emotions and being able to handle situations which arise in dating and learning how to handle their sexuality. Studies show that comprehensive programs, which teach both postponing sex and sex protection for those who decide to become sexually active, are more effective than any "abstinence only" programs and do not promote earlier or increased sexual activities.

The Netherlands, where sex education runs from preschool on, has the lowest teen birthrate in the world and their abortion rate is three times lower and AIDS rate eight times lower than ours in the U.S. Why don't we get it? Comprehensive sex education works best.

"Right Camp" sex education books carry blatantly false information: AIDS and STD's are the natural consequences of sex outside of marriage, STD's result in infertility, there are 100,000 new cases of syphilis a year, HPV's lead to vulvar cancer, condoms and contraceptives do not prevent disease and pregnancy, using condoms is very difficult, pre-marital sex causes mental illness, females who dress in an immodest fashion invite rape, and abortion is very unsafe. "Abstinence only" programs should be outlawed as unconstitutional, as they are promoting a religious agenda in public schools.Their views are certainly not true or believed by the majority, but in spite of this, they have managed to get federal funding since 1981 when Congress passed "The Chastity Law".

Taught properly by qualified instructors in a dignified and scholarly way, sex education may just create a positive, long-lasting attitude in our children. Students need to develop and internalize the idea that sex is a serious part of human life and not a recreational activity.

A new, effective sex education program called A PAUSE (Added Power and Understanding in Sex Education), based on extensive research at Exeter University focuses, not only on the physical side of sex, but on the emotional side. It combines the teachers presenting the technical aspects with input from peers and older teens. Peer educators (16-18 years) are given 25 hours of training and lead classes of 9th year students and mix role-play, media, and peer pressure to teach about sex and assertiveness techniques. Pupils at age 16, who have completed the course, are not only less likely to be sexually active, but are more able to cope with pressure to be sexually active. They are more prepared, when they decide it is right for them to become sexually active, to handle the physical and emotional aspects which arise. Any programs which attract and interest the young, increase their sexual knowledge, and delay their sexual activity are going to improve their chances of staying in school and their chances for a successful life.

HEALTH CARE
CHOICES

Two hundred years ago, or even one hundred years ago, the availability of health care was very limited so choice was hardly an issue. Regardless of whether you could get to a doctor or get a doctor to come to you, your choice was limited by the very few tricks he had in his little black bag. Today, with great increases in medical knowledge and equipment, that little black bag has become a trunk full of sophisticated drugs, miraculous diagnostic equipment, and modern hospital facilities. These advances can repair broken bodies and cure many complicated diseases. One would think that great choices abound. Unfortunately, today our choices in health care are still limited. They are limited by how much money you have. Employer provided health care insurance plans are a great benefit for those who have them, although many employers are increasing deductibles and co-payments in their health plans as a way to help combat rising premium costs. Insurance plans, at times, also restrict our treatment choices.

Closing Hymn. *p. 8 vs. 1.3.4*

VOLUNTEERS NEEDED! A bulletin board is located in Fellowship Hall with sign up sheets for activities that enhance our weekly church service and fellowship. Please consider volunteering for an activity that matches your interest.

vas diagnosed with breast can-
treatment at a cancer specialty
e of our insurance company's
ected to have her treated there
bout $17,000 in out-of-pocket
was not restricted because
pay for the choice we made.
estricted for someone who
My point in mentioning this
everyone should necessarily
tment through their insur-

ance. haps, our insurance company's preferred provider would have been just as good and our insurance company was just trying to keep premiums down by having their restrictions. The example is intended to illustrate that money does affect our choice in health care. We have all heard stories of people not receiving certain tests or treatments because they could not afford them and their insurance company would not pay for them.

Here is a specific recent example. It was a plea for help published in the letters to the editor section of a local newspaper. A single mother of two teens was diagnosed with aggressive Stage 3 breast cancer. She works in real estate sales to support herself and her children and has some health insurance. She is faced with the need to start fifteen weeks of chemotherapy as soon as possible. However, the chemo treatments are $4,600 each and she must pay $8,300 in advance before they will start administering them. Her insurance has a $5,000 deductible before they will cover her at 50% After chemotherapy, she faces surgery followed by twelve weeks of radiation treatments. She, like many working single mothers, just does not have the money to pay for all of this, even with insurance. A tragic situation.

If someone is under 65 and their employer does not have a health insurance benefit program, he or she must try to buy an individual policy. Many people cannot buy an individual policy because of pre-existing health conditions. When I retired before Medicare age, I lost my health insurance and, because of my employer's size, was ineligible for COBRA. I was unable to purchase health insurance because of a fairly minor heart condition. I don't blame the insurance companies for refusing me coverage. After all, insurance companies are not charitable institutions. They do not exist to help people. Their purpose is to make money. Their executives and shareholders expect them to make a profit. Nonetheless, it was a scary time for me. Luckily, I was eventually able to get coverage as a dependent under my self-employed spouse's plan.

Purchasing a private insurance plan can be a burden for many people. A man we know is a single father with two teenagers. He describes himself as "Joe Average". He works at two jobs and his health insurance premium is over $12,000 a year with a $5,000 deductible - per person - per calendar year. He feels that the cost of his health insurance is burdensome and that the high deductible is a form of health care rationing.

Forty-eight million Americans do not have health insurance. Some of those uninsured just don't want to bother with it. Some young adults feel invincible. Many more can't get insurance because of pre-existing conditions. Many, many more just can't afford it. We are told that the uninsured can always get care by going to an emergency room or negotiating with their doctor or hospital for free care or reduced rates. Recently, I took my wife to the emergency room because of a heart attack scare. After some tests, it was determined that it was a false alarm and, after spending three hours in the emergency room, she was released. The bill was over $4,000. Medicare covered it, but I wonder what degree of care and what tests she would have received if she had had no insurance or the means to write a check for that large amount.

On another trip to the emergency room a few years ago, a possible gall bladder problem was suspected and she was released and told to make an appointment with her doctor. Without insurance or the ability to fork over some cash, you usually won't get to see the doctor. You can't get past the guard at the reception desk without giving insurance information. You can't negotiate a fee with a doctor if you can't get in to see him. And, if you feel that hospitals won't go after you for unpaid bills, you are living in a dream world. I don't think that we should blame doctors for not giving free treatments. They deserve to be paid for their services. With that said, what do we do with our 48 million Americans who, for the most part, cannot afford health insurance? As a society, we have a choice. We can choose to say the heck with those 48 million fellow Americans or we can choose, as a society, to make some form of adequate medical care available to them. If we choose the latter, we can join all of the world's westernized industrial nations and have some sort or tax payer financed plan.

The health reform legislation, after a year of debate, became law in 2010. It is a start for reform, but falls short. It contains some taxpayer subsidies to smaller companies to cover up to 50% of their newly required health insurance premiums. It provides some government subsidies to lower income people for the purchase of private individual insurance plans. It also will give some help to seniors in the form of a rebate to fill part of the "donut hole" in the prescription drug program.

The law also includes some pretty silly sounding items, such as a 10% tax on tanning parlors and requiring chain restaurants to provide a nutrient content disclosure statement alongside their menu items. A tax on tanning parlors at the same time we continue to subsidize the growing of tobacco? Are we so delusional that we think a harried mother of four will take the time to read, much less understand or care about, a "nutrient content disclosure statement" while trying to supply her screaming kids with a lunch consisting of "Big Macs"? Talk about big brother's legislative overkill!

The 2010 health law does have some good features. Under it, insurance companies won't be able to drop a person because they get sick, not-for-profit health care organizations will need to maintain a medical loss ratio (money spent on benefits versus money coming in) of at least 85% to take advantage of their not-for-profit status with the IRS, and lifetime caps on the amount of insurance will be banned. Annual caps on benefits will be limited, and then banned in 2014, and also in that year, children will not be able to be denied health insurance because of pre-existing conditions. High risk pools are to be set up immediately to cover adults with pre-existing conditions and health care insurance exchanges will be established to eliminate the pools in 2014. In theory, these high risk adults with pre-existing conditions will then be able to obtain their health insurance coverage through the exchanges. Will these pools or exchanges be affordable? In fact, will any of it be affordable for the forty-eight million Americans presently without health insurance? The good parts of the new medical plan are bound to increase costs for insurance companies. That, in turn, has to increase premiums. The argument is made that, by forcing those who are healthier and have fewer claims to buy insurance, the insurance companies will be able to spread out their expenses and lower premiums. The jury is out on that.

For all of the impassioned rhetoric over the 2010 health law, I believe it is neither as good, nor as bad as critics have claimed. It will solve some problems, but it does nothing to reduce the cost of the health care which patients receive. There is much talk about government intervention, but whatever you call it, it is not socialized medicine. How can it be called socialized when we are getting it from private insurance companies, which are not controlled by the government? One can also ask, "How can the government order someone to use his hard-earned, after-tax money to buy a specific item from a private company"? It is true that states have the right to require a motorist to buy private auto insurance. That is done for the privilege of driving on a public road. One has the choice of declining to be a motorist and taking a taxi, bus, riding a bike, or walking to avoid buying that insurance. It seems that the 2010 health law requires every living person to buy health insurance. Are we really going to arrest, fine, and possibly jail Americans for refusing to buy a certain product from a private company? That will be interesting since there will surely be people who still absolutely can not afford to pay the premiums required under the new law. In addition to the presently uninsured, the 2010 health care plan will probably not be of much help to our friend, "Joe Average". He will still be paying premiums which he feels burdensome for coverage he feels is inadequate.

If we, as a society, want to chose something better than the status quo and feel that the 2010 health care law is not good enough, we will need to consider some government participation, which must imply some taxpayer consequences. The government's participation in paying for adequate medical care for all does not necessarily mean socialized medicine. Not that all socialized medicine is terrible. England's system of socialized medicine is certainly not perfect. Hospitals there are often crowded and many times there are long waits for elective procedures. We could say that their system provides care that is perhaps inferior to the care of those in this country who have good insurance or are wealthy, but better than the medical care available to our less fortunate fellow

Americans. Canada's health care system, although frequently maligned in the U.S., seems to work pretty well according to my many Canadian friends. Of course, no health system, including ours in the U.S., is perfect.

In the U.S., we have three distinctly unique health care programs in which our government is already involved. They are Medicare, Medicaid, and the V.A. system. Medicaid seems to be the stepchild of the three. It is means-tested and covers the poorest of our citizens, is managed by the states, is chronically under-funded, and pays so little to physicians that they are reluctant to participate in the plan. The government pays slightly more than half of Medicaid's cost with the balance paid from state budgets. I doubt if Medicaid could be extended from its present form to a universal program.

The Veterans Administration provides health care for our nation's veterans. I would call it our only true socialized medicine system. If one is eligible and chooses to participate in V.A. health care, one must accept V.A. doctors, V.A Hospitals, and V.A. treatments. In the V.A. system, all of a patient's records are in their computer system and may be accessed from any V.A. office, clinic, or hospital. Their system of keeping computerized health records would be a practical system for any comprehensive health plan. Instead of having easily accessible health records, when we go to a new doctor, we have to fill out reams of forms with our whole health history, and are advised of the patient's health privacy act. It seems that this obsession with "privacy" might very well lessen our ability to get a good, quick diagnosis in a life-threatening situation. At one time people with tuberculosis were removed from their families to a sanitorium for recovery in order not to cause the spreading of the disease. Not only is that not done today, the privacy act allows TB patients to frequent public places with no restrictions. Today, you and I are at greater risk from such communicable diseases because of the lack of restrictions on those who have them. Although the V.A. provides a valuable service, because of its limitations on patient choice, I doubt if a V.A.-type system would be acceptable to many Americans.

The third health care program involving our government is Medicare. It is limited to seniors over the age of 65. Some critics of the government and Medicare claim that Medicare is socialized medicine. They are wrong. Medicare is not socialized medicine. Although we pay a payroll tax during our working years to support Medicare (and social security), at age 65 we can choose whether or not to participate in the program. Almost everyone does sign on with Medicare since it has good benefits and an insurance company, if it would insure us at all, would charge extremely high premiums. If we choose to participate in Medicare, we will have a modest annual deductible and have to pay a monthly Medicare fee. In an effort to cover some of the escalating costs of Medicare, the monthly premiums have increased on a sliding scale based on income.

Under Medicare, we can go to the doctor, clinic, or hospital of our choice and Medicare will pay a pre-determined amount to the medical providers if they participate in the Medicare program. Medicare pays 80% of the allowable amount. The patient is responsible for paying the remaining

20% of the allowable amount. Many people buy private supplemental insurance to cover the 20% for which they are responsible. Almost all hospitals and clinics participate in Medicare. Some doctors do not. If we choose to go to a doctor who does not participate in Medicare, we will have to pay that doctor directly. Invariably, the charge is higher than the Medicare allowable amount. We can, however, get reimbursement for the allowable amount which Medicare would have paid the doctor by applying directly to Medicare.

Paul:

Several years ago, I went to a dermatologist who did not participate in Medicare. I went to her because I was very confident in her professional ability to handle my particular problem. After the procedure, I paid her directly and her office filed a Medicare form for me. I received a reimbursement check from Medicare in less than three weeks. It was for an amount less than I had paid the doctor, but that was what I expected. I made my choice in medical care and did not regret it.

Some people sign a yearly contract with and pay a fee to a "boutique" doctor, who will be available to them 24/7 and, in some cases, even make house calls. That type of arrangement is not covered by Medicare and must be paid for by the patient. That's fine. It is their choice, if they can afford it. I support the Medicare type government approach to health care. While I do not believe that government supported health care must provide "boutique" health care to everyone, the government can cover the cost of basic care for all. Those with the desire and financial ability, may upgrade to "boutique" doctors, private hospital rooms, and patent-protected drugs instead of generics. A private upgrade option should continue to exist.

I think a Medicare-for-all program would be a much better health care arrangement than the 2010 health care law provides. However, before such a Medicare expansion could be considered, it would be necessary to make a tough, realistic appraisal of Medicare, its current benefits, and funding. Two years ago, Medicare was predicted to run out of money by 2018. It may be able to last a few more years, but its financial position is precarious. Everyone in Washington D.C., Democrat or Republican, knows this. It is also common knowledge that the longer we wait to face the problem, the worse it will become. The solvency of Medicare is a much worse problem than that of Social Security and yet none of our elected officials will face the problem.

To solve Medicare's financial problems, several unpopular steps will need to be taken. People take advantage of large organizations. I have known people who pad or cheat on insurance claims because, "They are big companies and they can afford it", or, "Why not cheat, everyone else does"? The same is true of Medicare. People will go for a 2nd MRI or another EKG without questioning the real need, because Medicare will pay for it. Does the doctor own the facility where the test will be done? There may be a conflict-of-interest involved.

People will go to endless chiropractic appointments because Medicare will pay for them, but not go for massages which might also alleviate the problem, because they would have to pay for the massages themselves. A substantial, mandatory patient co-payment for each medical visit, to be sent directly to Medicare by the doctor when he sends for his Medicare reimbursement, would cut down on unnecessary visits. The co-payment could be on a sliding scale based on your last year's income tax return.

Figures indicate that one third of Medicare's expenses each year go for caring for patients in their last year of life and that aggressive care in the final months of life accounts for 80% of that. Except for the wealthy, care is rationed now by insurance companies, lack of insurance, and the hard reality of economics. If an insurance company says it does not cover a certain procedure, the patient has the choice of paying for it himself, or going without it. Whether or not we like the idea, the cost of caring for an aging population will require that we and our politicians accept the fact that we will need to ration health care at various times. Someday, Medicare will have to be prepared to say, "Sorry, but we do not pay for heart transplants for 80 year olds, we do not cover long-term ventilator care for terminal lung cancer, or brain-dead patients, and, we will not give you more chemotherapy because it will just make you feel lousy and it will not cure your cancer". A month in the hospital of no-holds-barred aggressive end-of-life care with no hope of living any longer or more comfortably could cost a half a million dollars or more. The alternative choice for the patient would be to opt for palliative care at home and leave that money in the system to care for those who have a chance for a long life. An interesting, unselfish, beneficent choice.

One of the hot buttons in medical treatment is the subject of medical malpractice insurance. Even though the medical community wins about 85% of the malpractice lawsuits which go to court, insurance premiums are high and often used by doctors to justify high fees. At times, smaller out-of-court settlements are made by insurance companies to avoid the expense of litigation. This situation is an irritant to the doctors who have to pay the high premiums and a significant source of income for the trial attorneys. Both can make good arguments to support their views on this subject. Doctors and hospitals will argue that approaches to treatments can vary, no medical treatment is risk free, people are human and can make mistakes no matter how hard they try, and some jury awards are way too excessive. The lawyers will argue that patients have the right to expect a reasonable standard of medical care and that doctors or hospital personnel should be held financially accountable for their professional errors, like elsewhere in our society. While some states have been able to pass caps on "pain and suffering" in medical lawsuits, such legislation is difficult to pass (so many legislators are attorneys) and it has failed to greatly reduce malpractice insurance premiums. Shouldn't a person who suffers greatly because of a blatant medical error be entitled to some financial recompense for his pain and suffering? How much money is enough, or too much?

What is the solution to this problem? The cost of insurance

premiums is burdensome to many physicians and many tests are performed not out of medical necessity, but for possible legal protection. Perhaps a partial solution to this problem could be achieved under a "Medicare-For-All" health program in which any doctor who participates would be legally freed from any financial claims due to medical malpractice litigation. This would increase the doctor's bottom line and be an encouragement to participate in the program. In conjunction with this, there would have to be a procedure for the filing of medical complaints which could lead to restricting the right of repeat or outrageous offenders to practice medicine. We could also give the patients the choice of buying an insurance policy for each procedure they undergo, which would allow them to file a suit for financial damages due to malpractice. The insurance company would be responsible for the payment of damages, not the doctor. Such a plan would be similar to the flight insurance people could buy before their air flight years ago. Patient choice - do you trust your doctor or not?

If a Medicare-For-All plan is instituted and a rather substantial co-payment charged for each visit to prevent people from abusing the system, our citizens will have to also be encouraged to exercise, eat moderately, and become knowledgeable about a bit of do-it-yourself medicine. Many over-the-counter generic drugs will relieve flu, cold, head, stomach pain, diarrhea, and ulcer symptoms without a trip to the doctor. An informational booklet for each family covering health issues and simple solutions which they can employ would save billions in Medicare costs, as well as creating a healthier society. Clinics staffed by LPN's , retired service medical personnel, and nurse practitioners would be able to treat minor injuries and illnesses at less cost, as well as take the burden from over-worked family practitioners who are in short supply. Doctors will have to cut back on expensive tests as much as possible. Now with a price tag of around $4,000, MRI's and CT scans are being done routinely, when less expensive tests would suffice. With all of the sophisticated tests available, a friend of mine spent eleven days in the hospital before they were able to determine that her gall bladder should come out. This was not an isolated incidence. Two other friends almost died when they suffered from a burst appendix. What's up with this? We both have refused to return for additional $4,000 tests when we felt that the need was really questionable even though, "Medicare would have paid for it". We made a choice of conscience regarding what we thought was a waste of taxpayer money. Perhaps, more people should do that, but if the people decide that they want to have every test that any doctor suggests, then the people as a whole will have to "step up to bat" and "pay the piper". Again, a matter of choice, both by the citizens of the country and by each person on an individual basis.

Barbara:
In my youth there existed a great quest for a "healthy, vibrant tan". My friends and I spent hours under tanning lamps, slathered with baby oil laced with iodine,

faces to the sun seeking the "perfect tan". Summers at the beach, tennis, boating without the benefit of UVA, UVB, titanium, or zinc oxide worked magic in creating the sun-damaged skin we now display with regret. In 1972, we moved to Florida to spend more time in the sun and soon skin cancers began to appear. My first dermatologist was Dr. A. He was all business and scraped and burned a spot on my nose - not fun, so I began to wear hats and sunscreen and tried a new dermatologist Dr. B. By that time ugly, dark, old-age spots were popping up everywhere. Dr. B. was friendly, but a bit cavalier in his approach. When I asked him to remove the dark, scaly spots that I didn't like, he told me that I could scratch them off. Started me thinking, but instead of scratching them off, which only made them red instead of brown and certainly wasn't a permanent solution, I decided to try another dermatologist. Dr. C. was recommended by some of my spotted tennis friends. He was great and would burn off 15 or 20 at a time and really seemed to care about his patients looks, as well as preventing future cancers by removing the brown, scaly, ugly pre-cancers.

Unfortunately, we had to change to Dr. D. when we lost our insurance and had to switch to a PPO. He was busier and limited his treatment to the number of spots our insurance would cover and always also wanted to do three biopsies (also the number our insurance covered). At four visits a year, three spots treated and three biopsies each visit, Dr. D. could make a lot of money and at the rate that suspicious spots cropped up, keep us coming forever at great cost to our insurance.

I am convinced, from our experience, that dermatology is often a "hit or miss" practice and that the interaction between Medicare/insurance coverage and the practice is not a good thing for patients. If insurance will pay for three biopsies, some doctors seem to be able to find three "suspicious areas" to biopsy, and only once in a dozen times did a spot turn out to be a cancer, and that was after I said, "Remove it" and the biopsy following the removal confirmed my concern. Every other time, I would get a call from the doctors office reporting that the biopsy was only "pre-cancer" and nothing had to be done about it at that time. Six months prior to the positive biopsy, I had pointed out that very spot and asked that it be removed only to be told by Dr. D that it was "nothing to be concerned about". The removal of the growth, left a great hole which took a long time to heal and then needed further treatment because of the scarring.

Paul:
While under the PPO and the care of Dr. D, I had a biopsy done on the side of my nose. The report came back negative. After the excised area had healed, it still looked odd, so back to Dr. D. who sent me to Dr. E. who did Mohs surgery. Mohs is a system which takes layer by layer in a series of small excisions, examining the tissue samples between excisions until no cancer cells are present. The idea is to save as much good tissue as possible. When cancer cells were no longer present, a whole area of my nose also was not present.

This necessitated three plastic surgeries which I believe could have been prevented by earlier intervention. The biopsy had possibly missed the small spot which could have been cut out when it was small, avoiding major reconstructive surgery and major cost. My example certainly points to the need for early treatment of all pre-cancers before they turn into full-blown problems. The present rationing system simply is not cost-effective nor does it benefit the patient. Another visit to Dr. E. resulted in five gaping holes in my legs with weeks of healing and treatment by my wife, who moaned that she didn't get paid for her time and changing my dressings wasn't her idea of a pleasant job. After the last session of sitting in Dr. E's waiting room with other patients and not enjoying the setting which looked like a scene straight from the operating room of the TV series MASH, I decided to try another dermatologist, again.

Recently a local dermatologist, who was doing unnecessary biopsies and surgery on his patients was sentenced to twenty-two years in prison. He had over-billed Medicare by seven million dollars which he is to pay back, as well as making restitution to over eight hundred patients who suffered needless surgery.

Barbara:
What is a poor patient to do? Skin cancer can be a killer and every patient is a potential skin cancer victim, but waiting until an area gets ugly enough to be "of concern"

to your doctor often calls for expensive, extensive, disfiguring surgery. If you develop new spots as quickly as I do and treatment is limited by your insurance, you are fighting a losing battle.

Feeling totally frustrated by the system and thinking about Dr. B's advice to "scratch them off", I began to experiment with "do-it-yourself dermatology". I had had enough spots removed by cryo-surgery to know how to do it myself, but couldn't obtain the liquid nitrogen needed to do it. Efudex is a cream which had been prescribed by one doctor and it does work by attacking fast-growing cells. The treatment takes at least two weeks and during that time there is a lot of stinging and itching as it turns pre-cancers from brown spots into red, raw, weeping spots. Then there is a slow healing process. The outcome is good, but cryo-surgery is faster and there is less extended agony. Liquid nitrogen is applied from a gun/canister or by a cotton swab dipped into the liquid nitrogen and then touched to the bad spot. The skin depresses and turns white. Later it turns red and sometimes develops blisters. The healing process begins right after and the skin must be kept clean and most doctors suggest the use of a topical antibiotic during the healing period.

What else would work the same and be available to a lay-person, I asked myself? I found that containers of a cold substance which warned you to only use it "on warts" would work, but they were a bit hard to control. I did treat many spots on my arms and legs that way with very good results. Although it was not as precise as professional cryo-surgery, the treatment and recovery were similar.

Finally, I hit on an easy, cheap, and effective way to treat pre-cancer spots . It was dry ice. I crack it with a hammer, hold it with a pot-holder and apply it to the spot. It depresses the skin and turns it white while freezing it, just like liquid nitrogen/cryo-surgery. It results in a burn or blister just the same and I treat the spots with an antibiotic ointment during the healing process, just the same as after professional treatment. I am informed regarding the signs of skin cancer and will seek professional treatment when necessary. I look better, have fewer spots waiting to turn into cancers, and avoid expensive trips to the dermatologist. Crazy? Maybe? My choice!

In the final analysis, a single-payer "Medicare-For-All" plan would probably have to adjust, and in some cases ration, benefits. It would need to discourage people from seeking treatment unnecessarily, through a co-payment for each visit. Doctors and patients will have to stop cheating. That will probably have to be strictly scrutinized because, unfortunately, I don't think that it is basically in peoples' general "human nature" to be honest. It will probably require additional tax revenues, but that will happen even if we do not adopt the "Medicare-For-All" plan. We can not keep getting more treatment for less money. The present Medicare program will run out of money in less than twenty years. The choices are ours.

CHOOSE YOUR POISON
ILLEGAL DRUGS

In the area of drug abuse, I again feel that the best choice for success in reducing our drug problem lies in the field of education. The U.S. Drug Enforcement Administration lists, under its "Programs and Operations", twenty separate categories. They range alphabetically from, "Asset Forfeiture" to "State and Local Task Forces". I am sure they all play an important part in the program to counteract the great costs to our nation due to illegal drugs and their usage. Programs have increased in number and cost as the population increases, but drugs have never been more prevalent, it seems, here and in other countries. Perhaps the DEA needs to step back and take a hard look at what is and is not effective and change their emphasis to those programs and methods which work best. They may have to cut out many ineffective programs and channel that money and effort into programs which reduce the drug problem.

In 1961, the DEA drug interdiction program was set up to cover plant-based drugs and in 1971 expanded to respond to the diversification of drugs to over one hundred additional, mostly synthetic, drugs. A further act of 1988 provided for comprehensive measures against drug trafficking. The results of several reviews, unfortunately, indicate that the increase in drug law enforcement intervention has not reduced drug problems or usage. There also has been an increase in violent crimes and homicides. These programs have not achieved the goal of reducing the drug supply.

There has also been a militarization of civilian SWAT teams with an estimated number of raids as high as 40,000 per year, resulting in many mistakes affecting innocent people and bystanders. Countries supplying illegal drugs simply are increasing their supplies to make up for seizures. Despite two years of extensive spraying with herbicides in Columbia, there has been no reduction in supply, in fact, coca growing has increased in that country. It is fairly clear that continuing the seizure of illegal drugs is not reducing the supply or use of these drugs.

The drug known as MDMA or Ecstasy is one of the most dangerous drugs threatening young people today and is one of the easiest illegal drugs to obtain. It has become very popular at concerts and parties, in spite of the severe penalties for possession, manufacturing, or delivery. Fines up to $100,000 and up to ninety-nine years or life in prison do not seem to eradicate the use of this drug, nor do the common side effects of sweating, nausea, anxiety, and increased temperature, blood pressure, and heart rate. The perceived increased confidence and feeling of well-being are enough reason for the user to take the chances of fines, incarceration, and even death. After just one use, the come-down is often severe enough to send the user for more to alleviate the depression, and that can lead to needing more and more until the habit can cost over $300 a day. The best solution in preventing such drug use is education. Most of what children and young adults hear about drugs such as ecstasy comes from those making money from selling them. That must change.

One group working to counteract the lure and glamour of drugs is the "Foundation for a Drug-Free World". They work to give young people facts which will, hopefully, lead them to the choice to lead drug-free lives. Educators and volunteers have distributed over 55 million handouts on drug education. It is necessary to reach the young with fact-based educational information before they start experimenting with drugs. Their education program consists of a documentary and thirteen booklets as well as award-winning public service announcements. The booklets have been distributed in over sixty countries and in twenty languages. It is easy to watch their dynamic documentary on the internet. It points out, by interviews with people who have been involved in drug use, the devastating effects various drugs have had on their lives. The work of the "Foundation for a Drug-Free World" is valuable and should be supported by any individuals interested in a drug-free world, as well as our government.

So education is, most acknowledge, a very important aspect in reducing the number of new users. However, educational deterrents do not reach all potential users before they try drugs and become dependent on them. In 1990, the U.S. Department of Education said that all public school districts were in compliance with the federal law requiring every public school to teach students that, "The use of illicit drugs and the unlawful possession and use of alcohol is wrong and harmful". It actually puts drug education courses in the position of being deemed "illegal" if they do not stress the aspect of drugs being "wrong" and in any way lead students to conclude that drug usage is a matter of choice. Apparently, some drug education courses are doing just that. Perhaps the problem of being in compliance with the statement comes from the fact that the statement lumps illegal drugs with alcohol, which is legal and can be used when a person is "of age". Choice must be allowed regarding substances which are legal, such as alcohol. Illegal drug use is wrong and harmful to individuals and society, in general. Therefore, there must be a differentiation between the use of illegal drugs and legal substances, such as alcohol.

What is the driving factor in the drug usage problem? It is money! The huge illicit drug industry makes great profits from creating need and drug dependency. It makes sense to attack the drug problem by reducing their market. How do we do this? I propose that in medium to large cities and other cities where drugs are prevalent, the government purchase large, cheap old hotels and apartment buildings. Either state governments or the federal government can implement this plan. I call these buildings, "Drug Zoos". In some of these buildings would be offered drug counseling and rehabilitation treatments for addicts who wish to "kick the habit" and return to society drug-free. Addicts who want to remain users would be housed in other "Drug Zoos". They would be provided with a room, food, and free drugs. Drugs would be dispensed from a locked cache and would have to be consumed in the addicts room. Food would be provided in a main dining room. The drugs would be easy to stockpile if authorities stopped destroying them and, hopefully, the need would dry up at the same time that the supply would dry up for lack of new customers. The value of street drugs would plummet. Drug lords, pushers and drug gangs would be out of jobs. Drug-related crimes would vanish. Incarcerations for drug possession and users would decrease. The cost of feeding and providing drugs to hopeless addicts would be a fraction of the cost we are now paying for all of our drug programs, and jailed users and addicts. The lure of, "trying a new drug for a great high" would be severely squelched if we included in our children's drug education classes, field trips to view the hopeless addicts in the "Drug Zoos".

CHOOSE YOUR POISON
TOBACCO

"In 1492, Columbus sailed the ocean blue". He stumbled upon the Americas and he and the conquistadors who followed him introduced the conquered native Americans to venereal diseases, small pox, chicken pox, measles, burnings at the stake, and slavery. In return, the native Americans introduced the European invaders to tobacco. Tobacco was carried back to Europe and eagerly embraced by the European populace. It turned out that, in the long run, the native Americans killed far more through their introduction of tobacco than did their invaders. After 500 years, the killings continue.

Tobacco associated deaths account for nearly one out of five deaths, or about 440,000 every year, in the United States alone. The number of yearly deaths caused by tobacco worldwide, where smoking is more socially acceptable, is staggering, 10,000,000 by some estimates. Although smoking can add to circulatory and heart problems, its main method of killing is through cancer. Pipes may primarily cause lip cancer, cigars and chewing tobacco may be contributors to mouth cancer, but the main organ which cigarettes attack is the lungs. There is nothing good or positive from suffering and dying from lung cancer. Death from lung cancer is painful and horrible. The only good thing regarding lung cancer is that it is largely preventable.

Barbara:

In 1956, as a senior in high school, I chose for my term paper thesis, "The Cigarette-Cancer Controversy". At that time, the facts which I was able to compile pointed to a definite correlation between cigarette smoking and cancer. Can you believe that after knowing what I had learned from writing that paper, I began to smoke at the age of twenty? I had never drunk coffee or smoked, and when I tried my first cup of coffee, which I didn't like, I decided to try a cigarette with it also. It was in a social situation and little did I think that I would get hooked. I smoked for 14 years and it was a maddening craving which I often regretted. I quit several times, even when we could buy cigarettes for $1.50 a carton, so the desire to quit was not influenced by the cost factor - as it would well be today. I enjoyed the cigarettes, but hated myself for smoking.

In the spring of 1972, my mom and dad visited us in Florida on their way back to Chicago. My mom had not been feeling well and went to the doctor on her return. A few weeks later, my dad called and said that they were going to remove my mom's one lung as they had diagnosed her with lung cancer. I took my package of cigarettes and threw it away and have never smoked another cigarette. I was with her when she died four months later. She had gone through a painful operation, nauseating chemo-therapy, and had attempted, unsuccessfully, to end her life to stop her suffering, only ending up in the hospital with more treatment. She was 56 years old when she died. I still miss her and wish that she had listened to the doctors who had advised her to quit smoking, before she developed the cancer which took her life.

In the early 1990's the tobacco executives testified before Congress, with straight faces, that the tobacco used in cigarettes was not scientifically proven to be injurious to one's health. They even produced bogus, misleading "scientific studies" to support their position in the same manner that global warming skeptics do today. Of course, the best way to lessen your odds of getting lung cancer is to make the choice to never smoke.

The tobacco situation in our present society is rather bizarre. Most people, even a lot of smokers, recognize the health dangers that go with smoking. There are about 44 million smokers in the U.S. today. This number is down from earlier years. Smoking has declined in our society because people have been made more aware of the health hazards, our government has increased taxes on tobacco products, and it has generally become socially unacceptable. Thirty years ago, no one would think twice about smoking a cigarette while a guest in someone's house. An ashtray was an important decorating item. Today it is hard to find an ashtray in most homes and smokers step outside on the porch or patio to light up a cigarette when at a party.

Non-smoking campaigns have existed for years. Our government first issued health warnings on cigarette packages in 1966. Yet, we continued to provide depression era quotas and price supports for U.S. tobacco growers until 2004. Public outrage over subsidizing tobacco growers resulted in the U.S. stopping subsidizing farmers through a system of price supports and quotas. The government bought the quotas and today farmers can grow as much tobacco as they want. It is their choice to grow tomatoes, turnips, or tobacco. The ten billion dollars being paid over a ten year period to the holders of the old tobacco quotas is being paid for by taxes on tobacco companies. I don't exactly follow the logic of paying ten billion dollars for old tobacco quotas and price supports which have been cash cows for their owners for seventy years. I always thought that all of our agricultural subsidies, including tobacco, were renewed and budgeted for annually and could be increased, decreased, or done away with entirely at that time. This is a good example of the wheeling and dealing and horse trading that goes on in Washington D.C.

Earlier in this book, we referred to Dr. Jack Kervorkian's belief that the Ninth Amendment to our Constitution should protect those who want to smoke in public. We don't agree with that assumption because second-hand smoke can surely be regulated as a matter of public health policy. It is important to realize that, when it comes to tobacco, people can choose to grow it or not and choose to use it or not. The former would be an economic decision. The latter could very well be a choice between life or death.

CHOOSE YOUR POISON
ALCOHOL

Alcohol is just one more substance which can get us in trouble. If used in moderation, it is said to be a possible health plus, but that amount is very small. Anything exceeding one beer, 4 ounces of wine, or 1 ounce of liquor transfers you into the negative health column. Alcohol is legal and taxed highly. Our country's experiment with the prohibition of alcohol was a flop. Probably the majority of people who choose to use alcohol do not have trouble with its use, but for those who end up with trouble using it in moderation, lives can be ruined. Some figures indicate that our country has 14 million people who would fall into the classification of being alcoholics. Alcoholism has been called "a disease", but that classification, in our estimation, gives a false "victim status" to the person who has become an alcoholic, making it harder for him/her to face their problem and quit.

Barbara:

My experience with using alcohol started in high school (illegally). It was something we did on dates, but never to excess. One exception was a girls pajama party when five or six high school friends and I decided to find out what it was like to "get drunk". We all kept drinking, danced around my friends basement, drunkenly laughing for hours - until we all got sick - "sick as dogs". When her parents came home, we said that the chili her mom had left us must have made us all sick. In later years, drinking was a part of parties and at times I would drink "too much" and get sick, always regretting the fact that I had drunk just too much - past relaxation, past fun, -to sick. My "sick experiences" finally caused me to develop a pretty good alarm system, which would set off a buzzer in my head which told me, "Switch to a soft drink". If alcoholism is a disease, I should have become an alcoholic. Both of my parents were alcohol abusers, if not alcoholics. Luckily, I developed my alarm system. I believe that people who become alcoholics have developed that dependency because they, unfortunately, have never developed an alarm system. At this age, I have gone from a moderate social drinker to a health drinker.

Alcoholism has become a prevalent social problem throughout the industrialized world. The more developed the countries, the more apt they seem to be to have increased numbers of problem drinkers and the related family and societal problems. With so many improvements in the past thirty years in health areas, the question arises, "Why do we still have so many alcohol abusers and why do we still suffer from the devastating effects of alcoholism"?

For the most part and for most people, "having a drink" is a social, pleasant experience. However, statistics on alcohol abuse indicate that a rather large number of people, about fourteen million Americans, abuse alcohol and should not drink. Over fifty percent of adults in the U.S. have an alcoholic in their family.

Medical research statistics show that alcoholism is extremely devastating to the alcoholic. It increases the risk for throat, colon, rectal, liver, kidney, pancreatic, and esophageal cancers. It damages brain cells and liver function and can harm a fetus. It is a major causative factor in vehicular deaths. Yet, in spite of all of these negative facts, most people ignore them or are ignorant of them.

In terms of cost related to alcohol abuse, it is estimated that such problems run about $200 billion per year. In terms of human lives, we must consider the costs of wasted lives, destroyed marriages, damaged children, illnesses, injuries, and deaths.

What is the answer to this societal problem? One obvious conclusion is that alcoholics, no matter where they fall on the progressive downward slide, need to get alcoholism information (again, education) and treatment. What educational information about alcoholism should be made available? Here are some facts which should be part of any education program:

- As high as forty percent of college freshmen binge drink - consuming more than five drinks at a party with half of those drinking more than ten to fifteen drinks.
- Every year more than 150,000 college students develop health problems related to their drinking.
- Recent figures show that sixty-two percent of high school seniors have been drunk within a six month period.

- Alcohol is the third leading cause of preventable death in the United States.

There is a difference between alcohol abusers and alcoholics. Alcohol abusers do not have the extreme physical and mental desire and need for alcohol that alcoholics have, but alcohol, nonetheless, negatively affects their lives. They neglect responsibilities at home and work, make impaired decisions, such as driving while drunk, and develop relationship problems.

An alcoholic has progressed to physical dependence and can not give up alcohol without experiencing physical and mental withdrawal symptoms: nausea, shaking, anxiety, and sweating. An alcoholic has an overwhelming need to drink and also a need to drink increasing amounts in order to feel the effects.

Because alcoholism has become such a prevalent problem, our country needs to develop a specific, effective education program aimed at young people before they become alcohol users. Alcoholism facts, information, and statistics have not been effective in reducing the numbers of people who develop this devastating, debilitating problem. The choice to abstain from alcohol use should be made to look as tempting and more beneficial than the choice to use it. It might adversely affect liquor company profits and government tax benefits, but people benefits would abound.

CHOOSE YOUR POISON
GAMBLING

Gambling statistics:

- 15 million people show some signs of gambling addiction.
- 37 states now have lotteries.
- The gambling business has grown tenfold since 1975.
- Gambling profits in casinos run 30 billion a year and lotteries add another 17 billion.
- Those with incomes under $10,000 bet almost three times as much as those with incomes over $50,000
- Gambling among young people is on the increase with even 14 year olds at 42%.
- There are now over 260 casinos in 31 states on Indian reservations.
- After casinos opened in Atlantic City, crimes within 30 miles increased by 100%.
- Internet gambling is growing at a rapid rate.
- The average divorce rate for gamblers is twice that of non-gamblers.
- The suicide rate is twenty times higher for gamblers.
- 65% of pathological gamblers commit crimes to support their gambling habit.

- Problem gamblers bet larger amounts, gamble more frequently, and spend more time per gambling session.

Signs of a problem gambler are:
- Inability to stop playing whether winning or losing.
- Preoccupation with gambling while neglecting work, family, and other responsibilities.
- Wide mood swings, restlessness and irritability while attempting to cut down on gambling.
- Use of alcohol, drugs, or sleep to escape.

Teen gambling can start off with a simple bet on "Who can do something better than the other", with no actual money changing hands, but can progress to the point of money, property, or services being forfeited by the loser. The legalization of casino gambling and internet gambling, along with the legal age to gamble in many states being 18, have contributed to increased teen-age gambling.

Gambling allure is being elevated by its being featured on TV poker shows. Poker popularity has experienced an enormous increase. The ease of on-line gambling, as well as the push to purchase lottery tickets, are making it easier to lose one's hard-earned money all the time. Lottery ads on TV abound and the friendly advice given in the ads, "Play responsibly", is ludicrous. I have a serious problem with government-sponsored ads encouraging the purchase of state-run lottery tickets. Getting hooked on buying lottery tickets can lead to serious gambling problems for some, but is taking away money needed for food and health care for many. In New York, a 2007 survey of teens estimated that as many as one-in-ten have a gambling problem. Anti-gambling education is being considered in many schools. Gambling is often linked with poor academic achievement and alcohol and drug use.

In spite of the negatives surrounding gambling, 63% of Americans approve of legalized gambling, 29% would favor banning or reducing it, and 22% say that is should be expanded. Gambling and crime often are associated, especially since many types of gambling are still illegal. When gambling restrictions were eased, criminals who had gambling savvy were the first to open up legal gambling casinos. Nevada casinos in the early years had clear links to organized crime, but improved their regulation at the mandate of the federal government, and today casinos are highly regulated and held to very high standards. Many casinos are publicly-held companies with shareholders and are under SEC scrutiny. They are licensed and regulated by the state governments as well. Other than the large casinos, there are many other types of gambling which are not as well regulated and are more accessible to organized crime. Gambling is a natural target for criminals because of the very large amounts of money which are involved. Gambling provides for the possibilities of skimming, money laundering, loan sharking, and kickbacks. Crime rates are significantly higher in cities which allow gambling.

Trying to determine whether gambling has a positive or negative impact on our economy is difficult because so many factors must be taken into consideration. It favorably impacts construction and leads to many jobs. Casinos need suppliers and staff, but social costs are difficult to determine and generally negative. Money spent on a gambling establishment is money which was in circulation and being spent elsewhere. Building and running casinos do not create wealth, they merely redistribute it.

Barbara:

Forty years ago, my husband had a business trip scheduled in Las Vegas. We had little money and transported a car out there for a dealer in order to save the cost of a flight for me. I had, I thought, devised a perfect scheme to win at Roulette and had put $100 aside to work my plan. Odds of red or black coming up would be 50/50 if there were no green spaces, but I figured that consistently betting red would turn red up in at least 1 in 5 or 1 in 6 times. By starting with a $1 bet and doubling it each time I lost, I would win $1 when red came up and then drop back to a $1 bet - slow, but sure. It worked for some time and I was slowly winning, $1 at a time, but sometimes having to wager $16 to win only one. Then, the impossible happened. I bet $1, black came up, $2, $4, $8, $16, and, $32. Black came up six times in a row. I was down $63 and didn't have $64 left to double again. So, I dropped back to $5 bets and bet six more times - six more blacks. I made two more small bets - two more blacks - my money was gone. Black had come up fourteen times in a row. It was a black day for me, but a lesson which ended all the excitement of gambling and any desire to do it again. In my whole life, I have bought only one lottery ticket. Recently, a Texas woman won her fourth lottery. It was worth 10 million dollars. Her previous three wins were for 5.3 million, 2 million and 3 million. She'll probably keep betting. Who said life was fair?

Lotteries have been prominent throughout history and in modern times were reintroduced by the state of New Hampshire in 1964. Lotteries, along with their close cousin BINGO, are still the most popular forms of gambling. Arguments against lotteries include their symbolizing the boredom and materialism of life today and preying on the poor and uneducated. Supporters argue that it is a painless tax, with money being raised for good causes through people having fun. I, for one, do not think that it is fun to lose money, but that is a matter of choice - your choice.

CHOOSE YOUR POISON
MARIJUANA

In 1937, the Marijuana Tax Act was passed, levying taxes on anyone associated with cannabis, hemp, or marijuana use, sale, or possession. Violators could face up to $2,000 in fines and 5 years imprisonment. In 1951 a new marijuana act was passed criminalizing the possession and use of cannabis, hemp, and/or marijuana. In 1970 the Controlled Substances Act listed cannabis/marijuana as a Schedule 1 drug. In spite of that act, many states and cities have decriminalized marijuana, making use and sale low priority offenses. Although many attempts have made to take cannabis/marijuana off the Schedule 1 list, the Supreme Court ruled in a 2005 decision that the federal government has jurisdiction over the legal status of marijuana.

The U.S. prison population is six to ten times higher than that of most Western European nations. This is in great part due to the emphasis the Drug War places on arresting people on marijuana charges. Since 1990 almost six million people have been arrested on marijuana charges. In 2000 over 700,000 were arrested on marijuana violations.

Marijuana is in most cases used as "a recreational drug of choice" and research seems to indicate that it does not cause the problems which alcohol causes. In some cases it is used medicinally. The question exists and has been bandied about for some time, "Should we, as a country, legalize marijuana"? Those who favor legalization say it causes no deaths by its use, while legal drugs cause 20,000, alcohol 100,000, and tobacco 400,000 deaths a year. They claim that politicians and prohibitionists have for the past fifty years, made false claims, given incorrect statistics, and peddled scare stories to keep marijuana from being legalized.

The Division of Alcohol and Drug Abuse Web site says that the amount of THC, the psychoactive ingredient in marijuana is as much as ten times that of the marijuana used in the 1970's. That is refuted by those who favor legalization. Other DEA assertions are that marijuana has more cancer-causing agents than tobacco, can cause chest pains because of increased heartbeat, and slows reflexes and thinking which causes a definite danger on the highways. Because marijuana use often is combined with alcohol and tobacco use (both legal and taxed), it is hard to allocate degrees of blame.

Like any substance, marijuana can be abused. It can cause lethargy and short term memory loss while under the influence. Long-term use can cause bronchitis, but that effect can be eliminated by ingesting it. A 1997 UCLA study on 243 smokers over an eight year period reported the following: "Findings from the long-term study of heavy, habitual marijuana smokers argue against the concept that continuing heavy use of marijuana is a significant risk factor for the development of chronic lung disease" "Neither the continuing nor the intermittent marijuana smokers exhibited any significantly different rates of decline in lung function when compared with those who never smoked marijuana". The study concluded: "No differences were noted between even quite heavy marijuana smoking and non-smoking of marijuana".

The National Institute on Drug Abuse, Bureau of Mortality Statistics site states that marijuana does not cause serious health problems like tobacco and alcohol, such as strong addiction, cancer, heart problems, birth defects, liver damage, and emphysema. Searching "marijuana addiction" on the Web, however, shows many sites offering to help people get over their addiction to marijuana, so obviously users or friends and family of users must think that it causes problems. The use of marijuana does not seem to lead to the use of more addictive drugs.

The Netherlands' drug policy is the most non-punitive in Europe. For more than twenty years citizens of legal age have been able to buy and use marijuana in government regulated coffee shops. Their policy has not caused a dramatic escalation of usage and the Dutch approve of their current policy.

If marijuana were legalized in the U.S., billions of dollars would be saved in enforcement, legal and prison costs. Over five hundred economists have said, "It's time for a serious debate about whether marijuana prohibition makes sense". The Marijuana Policy Project in Washington D.C. admits that they know that prohibition has not kept marijuana away from kids, since year after year 85% of high school seniors tell government survey-takers that marijuana is "easy to get". While it is not entirely safe, its dangers have been overstated. Legalizing it would not convince us to even try it, but at the present time, the choice to use marijuana can result in severe legal penalties. Your choice!

A CHOICE OF BEHAVIOR

Barbara & Paul:
It seems that uncivil behavior has been steadily increasing during our seventy plus years on this earth. Our families expected polite behavior from us, as well as did our teachers. We were taught to say "please" and "thank you" and to respect all elders. Neither of us attended private or religious schools and the public schools we attended neither displayed the Ten Commandments nor had a prayer time at the beginning of classes. Even the "Pledge of Allegiance" did not have the phrase, "under God" at that time, but we respected our teachers and were shamed if we talked out of turn or disrupted the class by "being put out in the hall". That was usually enough punishment to make us "straighten up". Oh, for the good old days!

Now we see children being uncivil to their peers, parents, and teachers, and adults have followed right after, emulating their two year olds temper tantrums. When we first came up to our condo in the N.C. mountains in 2004 with our granddaughters, ages seven and four, we decided not to hook the TV cable up. We were sick, sick, sick of the rude pre-election political shenanigans. It had become impossible to understand the content of the programs because of the rudeness of the participants. So called "talk programs" had become "shout programs". This is our 7th summer without TV and it is blissful. Time to read, write, golf, paint, hike and just think. We do get one weekly news magazine and enough current news from the computer to fill our "need to know". We catch up with FOX, MSNBC, and CNN while on the treadmill at the recreation center.

When did all the incivility begin? Politics have become particularly ugly and politicians no longer seem to be able to discuss the issues without smearing their opponent. Unfortunate, as there are lots of serious issues facing our country which really need to be civilly "hashed out". Instead we have our politicians shouting down their opponents, making false accusations, and using character assassination. When Congressman Joe Wilson shouted, "You lie" at our president, he got loads of press plus a million dollars from rude supporters of his rude behavior. The resolution "to disapprove" his behavior failed. A sad commentary on our political situation.

Sports heroes have become rude and immoral, showing a complete lack of respect for others. Only the scenario of, "I win - you lose" is acceptable to them. How commonplace swearing and rude gestures have become when a player disagrees with an umpire's call. Screaming obscenities and taunting has replaced good sportsmanship in competitive sports. Examples of this "I win - you lose" attitude are also rampant in corporate America where those in control play out their agendas to gain wealth at the expense of anyone they can cheat. What is fair, just, and civil is, "Out the window".

Some of our electronic convenience devices have gone from not only causing us to behave poorly in our interaction with other people, to actually being life-threatening. We have always referred to call-waiting as "call- rude" and would never use it. Answering machines can be polite and helpful with a pleasant message which treats the caller as a person of worth. Cell phones can be used positively in emergencies or worthwhile situations, but having cell phone addicts prattle on in public places about their private life or inane subjects is rude to those around them. Distracted driving because of cell phone use or, worse, "texting" led to 5,474 vehicular deaths last year - one out of every six traffic fatalities, and another 448,000 people were injured. One study by Car and Driver showed that a driver, when legally drunk, took 4 feet longer to stop in an emergency situation, 36 feet longer when reading an email and 70 feet longer when sending a text.

Having good manners does not come naturally to people. It is a skill which not only must be taught to the young, but must be reinforced throughout our lives. Most of our lessons came from our parents and teachers. Parent and teacher influence now makes up a far smaller segment of the learning experiences of the young. Much of the children's time in their formative years is now spent watching TV programs which have little moral value and are rife with sex, violence, and rude behavior. No wonder we are seeing cruel, rude children as the result.

Manners, or a code of behavior in social situations, are necessary when there is a community in which you live. If you live alone, in the woods, never coming into contact with other human beings, you can do whatever you want to, if you do not affect others negatively. Etiquette predates law and is necessary in a community to keep people from killing each other. There have been rules of etiquette throughout history. Every society must have these rules. The Bible is full of rules which are really rules of etiquette. Etiquette depends upon those who practice it and has only the punishment of social disapproval to enforce it. Therefore, it is not the same as immoral, punishable behavior.

The attribute which most distinguishes the politics of a civil society is civility which is described as: caring for the interest of the whole society; having a strong desire for the common good. When conflict arises, a civil person is called to consider the greater common good versus personal or family gain. The problem of order in society arises because there is an inherent conflict between the desires of individuals and the requirements of a civil society. Our aim must be to reduce strife and establish civil discourse which can make possible the pursuit of our common goals. Without civility, it would hardly be possible for a society to exist at all. If there is no civil society, a totalitarian society is "waiting in the wings".

Groups, political parties and associations are necessary as intermediaries between individuals and the government in a civil society. Individuals, through their association with political parties and various interest groups, strive to influence government decisions in areas which will affect their lives. When incivility is rampant, reason and pragmatism disappear in our discourse. The Honorable Clarence Thomas has written, "Indeed, it has become almost (a) cliché of late to observe that civility is disappearing from public discourse and public conduct", and fears that, "Unless each of us, whether as judges, lawyers, professors, students, or citizens, encourages others, by example, to become more civil, we will be contributing to the erosion of the rules that allow our civil society to function".

Since the propriety of displaying the Ten Commandments in schools and public places is disputable along with prayer in schools, due to their religious character, how about a new non-religious "Ten Commandments of Behavior"? Here are some suggestions:

1. PAY ATTENTION: Pay attention to what is going on around you. Act thoughtfully in how you relate to the people around you when driving, talking to or about people and talking on cell phones.

2. BE CAREFUL: Be careful in your appearance and in how you treat others and their property.

3. ACKNOWLEDGE OTHERS: Acknowledge all people with a pleasant greeting. Do it first.

4. SMILE: Needs no explanation.

5. SHOW INTEREST IN OTHERS: Be empathetic. Put others first.

6. LISTEN, LOOK, LEARN: Be open to new experiences and knowledge.

7. BE POLITE: Use pleasant language, Please, Thank you and Excuse me.

8. THINK THE BEST: Think the best of others and of yourself. Seek to build others up.

9. RISE TO THE OCCASION: Seek excellence in all things.

10. BE PART OF THE SOLUTION: Be part of the solution to problems - not part of the problem.

Try choosing to follow the Ten Commandments of Behavior and see if civility isn't catching. You can even post them in a public place!

CHOOSE YOUR
WORDS CAREFULLY

Barbara:
When I was a child, during the WWII years, I lived with my mother, aunt, and two great-aunts. Two of the four were English teachers. There was an 18" hard rubber ruler applied to my backside for really misbehaving. Luckily that only happened a few times which I can remember - the fear of the "druller" was enough to keep me in line. Those four women plus some really good grammar school teachers made me learn and appreciate when to use I/me, she/her, he/him, they/them, and we/us. It really isn't too hard to do, but every day in every way we hear the use of those pronouns mangled. We also learned how to diagram sentences which taught us when to use adjectives and when to use adverbs. We also learned when to properly use the verbs is/are and was/were. How often do you hear, "I played good", instead of, "I played well"? Why aren't these language skills taught today, or are they glossed over and then just ignored? Poor speech is a large part of the "dumbing down of America". It is hard to believe that proper use of English has been taught in our schools for years, since there is not a newscaster who employs it. One of my "pet

116

peeves" is the use of "There's" all of the time. "There's" is a contraction of the words there and is. "Is" is a verb which requires the use of a singular subject or object, such as, "There's (there is) a flower in the garden". Why do we hear, "There's flowers in the garden", "There's boats on the lake", "There's dogs in the park", etc.? It seems that the proper usage of the words "there are" or the contraction, which is a bit cumbersome, "there're" has been completely lost. The same goes for the use of "where's". It also should only be used with a singular subject or object. Is it so much easier to say, "Where's the boys"?, than, "Where are the boys"? Bring back the word "are".

Political/gender correct English:

Lately, our choice of words has been influenced by political correctness, particularly in the gender area. Have you noticed how the word "man" has been gradually erased from our vocabulary? "Person" or "human" have been substituted for "man". "Man" and "mankind" have been used to signify the human species (homo-sapiens), as distinguished from other forms of life, throughout the ages and as early as biblical times, (Genesis 1:27). Man and mankind encompass male and female. Yet, apparently, some people feel these terms are sexist or gender-biased and we have been encouraged to "do away with man" and substitute "humankind" for "mankind". Not only is it more cumbersome to say "humankind" than "man" or "mankind", it really does not solve the problem. The politically correct "humankind" still includes "man". To carry this gender-bias mania further, it would be logical to substitute "Hupersonkind" for "humankind" and thus get rid of the dreaded "m" word. However, upon further study, we find that "hupersonkind" would still be lacking in gender neutrality since it contains the word "son" in it. The word "son" is obviously masculine and, therefore, probably unacceptable to the gender gendarmes. Perhaps, we should substitute "it" for "son" and make reference to "huperitkind" instead of "hupersonkind". After all, "it" is certainly one of the most gender neutral words we have, isn't it? It's a guess where this person/human nonsense will lead. I hope the craze does not extend to surnames. Somehow, I just can't see me referring to our 33rd president as Harry S. Truperson or Truperit.

The Past Past Tense:

Another annoying hack-job on our English language occurs in the telling of stories. Using the past tense has become a thing of the past. We hear our news in the present tense, although it happened an hour ago, yesterday, a week ago, or even years ago. Some present tense story telling is done to create excitement and to transport the person listening to the scene, but, "The police shoot the victim" is not exciting to me - it's stupid. The police shot the victim (even one minute ago) is the correct way to report an incident. I lose the whole train of a news story by having to correct the verb tenses while listening. Even historical documentaries, which I generally enjoy, are trying to use the present tense and often they flop back and forth between tenses creating utter confusion for themselves and their listeners. It is my hope, and may be my dying hope, that our story-tellers and newscasters will again, choose the past - the past tense.

The "F" Word (filler word):

There are some words which clutter our language incomprehensibly. The most common offenders are, "err", "uh", "um", "you know", and the rampant "like"/"was like" which most often replaces the word "said" in the stories of our grandchildren; "So, I was like, "No way", and she was like, "Yes, really". The word "like" is also just stuck in for no apparent reason. "Mom, like I really want to go to the store". The "F" word which was considered in really bad taste when we were young is now so common-place in common people that they can hardly speak without interspersing the "F" word once or twice in each sentence. Movies use it often, although it is still bleeped out on TV, and is f...ed out in newspapers.

We all have choices in the words we use. They affect our ability to interact, influence, and achieve. Choose your words carefully.

ANNIE GET YOUR GUN

The Democratic party has, with a stated goal of reducing crimes and homicides, introduced the "Gun Control Act of 1968", the "Brady Bill of 1993", and the "Crime Control Act of 1994". Their favoring gun control may have turned rural voters against them in 2000. The only gun issue on the 2008 platform was that of possibly renewing the 1994 "Assault Weapons Ban". A bill to renew the "Assault Weapons Ban" and make it permanent was introduced in Congress in 2008, but it died in committee.

Gun control is an intensely debated choice issue. Most gun related violence is found in poor rural or urban areas. The Center for Disease Control and Prevention (CDC) estimated that there were 65,000 gunshot injuries in the year 2000. The majority of deaths from guns in the United States are suicides, with almost 17,000 occurring in 2004.

Gun policy in the U.S. hinges on the interpretation of the highly debated Second Amendment to the Constitution which states, "A well regulated militia, being necessary to the security of a free State, the right of the people to keep and bear arms, shall not be infringed". The Supreme Court took the position in 2008 that the Second Amendment did secure an individual's right to own firearms. It was, however, actually a fairly narrow holding in that the judges specified that some local controls regarding possession in certain public places by individuals such as felons or mentally disturbed people, etc. could be enacted.

During the 1980's and early 1990's, homicides, primarily using handguns, increased greatly, reaching as high as 14,000. Homicides with knives, on the other hand, exceeded 4,000. The homicide rates in the U.S. are two to four times that of other developed countries.

The right to own a gun and defend oneself is considered by some as important to our identity as Americans. This feeling stems from our frontier history, as guns were necessary in our westward expansion. Guns were needed by the early settlers for defense against "bad men", foreign powers, unfriendly natives, and wild animals. Early settlers were responsible for much of their own protection and procuring of food.

As we have grown older, our perception of our personal need to own a gun has changed. We bought a gun in the 60's because we felt threatened living in an area prone to violence. Luckily, nothing happened and we never needed to use it. Now we live in a safer place and avoid situations and locations prone to violence. Some people can not avoid dangerous situations because of their occupations. They may feel the need to carry a weapon. The spread of concealed "Carry Laws" since 1986 has led to the widespread carrying of concealed handguns by civilians in many parts of the United States. We can't foresee our need to ever take our handgun out of our house and would be happy to never need to use it.

We can understand someone wanting to keep a shot-gun or rifle for hunting purposes, keeping a handgun in their home for self-protection, or even carrying a weapon while working in risky occupations in dangerous areas. We are, however, bothered when we read of a mother packing a gun while attending her child's soccer event, or see someone wearing a sidearm at a political rally. We are troubled when we see that one state has allowed guns to be worn in bars (what a recipe for disaster) or when we read how another state has passed a law specifically allowing employees to bring a gun to work (to be left in their car, if their employer objects to it in the workplace). We are con-stantly reading about gun abuses - from mass shootings to the shooting and killing of a teenager by an irate motorist whose car was hit by an egg on Halloween.

The National Rifle Association is a champion of unfet-tered, unregulated gun ownership, even automatic weap-ons. To us, that is an unconscionable position. Automatic weapons are good for one thing - killing people, lots of them. They are not necessary for protection within one's home and they are not used for hunting. As that stalwart conservative, the late Barry Goldwater said in 1990, "I am completely opposed to selling automatic weapons. I don't see any reason why they ever made semi-automatics. I've been a member of the NRA. I collect, make and shoot guns. I've never used an automatic or semi-automatic for hunting. There's no need to. They have no place in any-body's arsenal". So much for any "sportsman's argument" in support of automatic weapons.

The Supreme Court has upheld the right to, "keep and bear arms", but subject to reasonable controls, much like the right to free speech. The question for us is: Does widespread gun ownership cause or prevent crime, violence, and death, and should we press for reasonable restrictions (like we do in free speech)? Your personal opinion and ideas on this subject will affect your choice.

AN EMOTIONAL CHOICE ISSUE

Information gleaned from Wikipedia relates that same-sex marriage is most often based on human rights issues, mental and physical health relationships, and equality under the law. There are financial, psychological, and physical health benefits to children being raised by two parents in a government-recognized union. Policies which bar such unions are based on the "sanctity of marriage" and "stigma of homosexuality". There are presently at least ten countries acknowledging same-sex marriage. Mexico allows it only in Mexico City, while the U.S. allows it in at least six states. It is recognized, but not performed in five countries and four U.S. states. "Civil unions" are recognized in twenty additional countries, as well as performed in some jurisdictions in four additional countries and nine U.S. states. Forty-six additional countries, as well as twenty-one of our states are in current debate regarding this issue. It is certainly at the forefront in current governmental issues world-wide.

For most of recorded history, marriage has been a term which denoted a legal bond between one man and one or more women. A woman often did not have any choice in the matter, and in some countries and cultures this is still the case. The 1922 edition of "The History of Human Marriage" defined marriage as, "a relation of one or more men to one or more women which is recognized as custom or law and involves certain rights and duties" for the individuals who enter into it, and any children born from it. This definition failed to recognize same-sex marriages which have been documented around the world, including in more than thirty African cultures. The Oxford English Dictionary has recognized same-sex marriages since 2000.

In some instances, due to religious beliefs, marriage is also considered a sacred commitment a man and a woman make to each other in front of a religious leader and allowed by law. People who remain single in our culture have the choices of continuing to live with parents or one parent (if the parents consent), with another person either of the same sex or the opposite sex, with a group, or alone. Because it was so commonplace, a term for an unattached opposite sex pair living together was even coined -POSSLQ (persons of the opposite sex sharing living quarters).

The government has chosen to give certain financial benefits to married couples. We must ask the question, why does the government give financial benefits such as: tax breaks, marital deductions, joint-filing breaks, deductions for dependents and social security benefits for surviving dependent partners and children? Are these benefits given to promote the "traditional family"? Same-sex couples who want to be bound to each other legally are asking for the same type family benefits. If our society legalizes same-sex unions and there is no rational reason to withhold monetary benefits, it seems that the same benefits should accrue to those legal same-sex unions. This decision will have far-reaching monetary effects. If the government decides that these benefits only apply to the "traditional family" then same-sex couples would not be treated the same as opposite-sex couples in regards to tax benefits. The government must choose what type unions it will allow and what benefits will be allowed to these various types of "family units".

Being from what would be termed a very "traditional family" - married 52 years, two children, two grandchildren, we feel that the term "marriage" should be reserved for the traditional union of opposite sex couples. Same sex unions, if sanctioned by individual states or the federal governments, could have some other designation, such as "civil unions".

If same-sex unions become legalized by our government and all benefits given to traditional families are extended to those in legal unions, a further problem may arise. What would prevent any two people from creating a "civil union" solely for the purpose of obtaining tax benefits? This would be a much different situation from giving tax benefits to a committed, loving same-sex couple raising children.

Many have suggested that reserving the word "marriage" for religious, male/female unions and "civil unions" for same-sex unions would strengthen the separation between church and state and that mixing up the term "marriage" with contractual agreements is a threat to "traditional marriage". It is an emotional issue, but demands our consideration. How shall we choose?

TO SUE OR NOT TO SUE

Barbara:

I hope that there will never be a time in your life when you have to make the choice, "Shall I sue or not"? Twice I have been faced with that question of whether or not to seek recourse against an individual who caused me injury and extensive, lasting pain.

The first injury was from a car accident in which there was no question of any fault on my part. I was twenty-three. My husband, child and I had just gotten back home to Chicago after his three years of army service. We had no insurance, as he had just started his new job and there was a three month waiting period before our insurance kicked in. We had one car and I did not work, as day care and transportation would have taken almost all I could earn. My mother had had some surgery and needed help, so my husband dropped me and our baby off at my parent's house to care for her. She needed some medication so, with the baby napping, I took her car to go to the pharmacy. While at a stop light making a hard right turn, I was rear-ended by an old man traveling at 45mph. I had a torn left shoulder and a severe neck whiplash injury (before headrests). Getting the medical care I needed was difficult and expensive. A friend's father insisted that I see a

127

fellow attorney who could help me with getting my medical cost covered and a possible settlement for a probable long-term situation. He took my case which went on for years and necessitated difficult trips downtown to see the attorney and for depositions. The old man died before the case was settled and I remember receiving $400.00 as a settlement - hardly enough to cover my early bills and certainly not adequate to cover future bills I had for ongoing neck pain, much less any compensation for the pain. The good news is that old age and arthritic bone spurs have, in time, fused my neck to the point that the bad pain has mostly disappeared.

At fifty-five, I fell off a two story roof (definitely my fault), but my medical care was so poor that I now suffer a lot of pain daily and will as long as I live. I was taken by ambulance to the hospital with excruciating pain in my mid-back. The only diagnostic procedure done was an x-ray of my back which was of very poor quality and therefore hard to read. I could not move or get out of bed because of the pain. At day 3 the specialist, whom I had seen before for my neck pain, came in (according to the charts) and said the x-ray was misplaced and they were trying to find it. On day 6 he came in and told me that my injury was not any worse than an 85 year old woman stepping off a curb and used the word "inconsequential" three times. He told me I should get out of bed. I asked if he could get me a brace to help me. He said that I could ask my family doctor for a brace if I thought that I needed one. I did get my family doctor to order a corset for me and they lashed me into it and dragged me out of the bed up onto my feet. The pain was unbelievable. At day 10, I was released from the hospital, never having had a follow-up x-ray or a MRI or CAT scan which would have shown a severe break of the T-8 vertebra. That break, which with proper treatment might have had a chance to heal, led instead to the complete collapse of my T-8 vertebra and the compression of my spinal canal and spinal cord by one third. Any attempt to fix it surgically, after the collapse was noticed in a six week lung x-ray, held a significant chance of paralysis and a small chance of diminishing the pain significantly. My brother, an orthopedic surgeon in California, said that it was a, "Slam dunk malpractice case and that a first year intern should not have made such a mistake".

Not being able to get a local attorney to handle a case against a local doctor, we had to drive 70 miles to see an attorney who agreed that I had received terrible medical care from "Dr. Inconsequential" and that he deserved to be sued. He, however, advised us that if he were to take the case for me that I might be compromised in my eventual ability to function by not being able to pursue the strenuous exercise program advised by the Miami Spine Institute. In other words, my working to try to regain strength and function would be detrimental to any eventual settlement. In addition, he told us that the doctor would probably be able to find an "expert witness" who would say that, even if the break had been discovered and treated, there would have been a chance that it "could" have still collapsed.

Since my desire to sue was driven by the pain I experience daily, along with the lousy medical treatment and care I received from "Dr. Inconsequential", more than the desire to get money, I decided not to bring a lawsuit against him. I hope he became a more effective and caring doctor after he found out how serious the outcome of his flippant attitude and pathetic practice of medicine were to me. He found out when my family doctor sent him a copy of the lung x-ray report, done at six weeks, showing the seriousness of my condition. When my husband called his office three months after the accident to inquire about why we had not received his bill for my hospital care, he was told, "There was no charge for the doctor's services" How strange! My experiences regarding suing for real injury where there was no fault on my part probably influences my attitude regarding lawsuits of any kind - both just and unjust. I am, no doubt, less empathetic than most people when it comes to people suing over minor injuries and trivial grievances. I say, "Choose to get over it, get on with your life, pick up your feet, look where you are going" A huge monetary settlement in either the case I pursued or the case I did not pursue would not have resulted in my experiencing less pain from the injuries I sustained. In fact, if I were able to turn the hands of time back and avoid the pain I have experienced, I would be willing to pay a great deal. But, that is a choice I will never have.

Regarding the law in general, there has been much discussion bandied about regarding "tort reform". "Frivolous" is also used to describe lawsuits where there is only a bare connection between the action of the defendant and the injuries of the plaintiff or where the plaintiff is seeking damages which are viewed as excessive for the injuries sustained. Tort reform supporters also cite lawsuits based on cases where the plaintiffs have suffered absolutely no tangible harm or where harm can be blamed on the negligence or irresponsibility of the plaintiff. Proponents of tort reform say that frivolous lawsuits are common and costly.

In the healthcare field, tort reform advocates want to impose caps on non-economic losses and punitive damages as well as set limits on "contingent fees". They argue that caps would benefit plaintiffs with legitimate lawsuits by reducing "nuisance" suits, making the system more efficient, especially concerning personal liability and class action suits. On the opposite side of the issue you find those who argue that, including legal fees, insurance costs, and payouts, the cost of all medical malpractice suits comes to less than 1% of all health care spending. They feel that medical malpractice pressure results in better care for patients. It is reported that there has been a great drop in medical malpractice insurance premiums for doctors in states which have enacted tort reform, particularly in those who capped non-economic damages.

In other areas, tort reform supporters point out that reforms can make significant cuts in the cost of doing business which may be passed on to customers. The cost of product liability can be so high that innovation is squelched. They allege that our present day approach exceeds any reasonable need to protect consumers. Critics contend that proposed changes would shield large corporations from having to pay just compensation for damages to consumers. In the case of the over 3,500 homeowners whose homes were built using tainted Chinese drywall, there was no direct legal recourse available to them against the Chinese manufacturers or the unsuspecting builders in most cases. In April 2010, a federal judge awarded 2.6 million in damages to seven Virginia families for Chinese toxic drywall damages, but will they ever be able to collect one penny from the Chinese manufacturers? This is a tragic instance of poor control of imported items and not the only one. Thankfully, the IRS has just made the decision to allow tainted drywall victims to claim a casualty loss deduction to help them cover the cost of repairing the damage to their homes.

We hear much about class action lawsuits. They have the advantage of combining many similar cases into one lawsuit worthy of an attorney's labor. A defendant who causes widespread harm, although of minimal monetary value against each individual plaintiff, will have to compensate those individuals for their injuries. Also, class action suits are used to change the harmful behavior of a defendant or class of defendants. The preamble to the Class Action Fairness Act of 2005 passed by Congress stated, "Class action lawsuits are an important and valuable part of the legal system when they permit the fair and efficient resolution of legitimate claims of numerous parties by allowing the claims to be aggregated into a single action against a defendant that has allegedly caused harm. A major criticism is that class action plaintiffs often receive little or no benefit from class suits due to large attorney's fees and confusing information regarding their rights.

Lawsuit abuse has removed many useful products from the market place and added costs to many other products.

Lawsuits have caused the maker of Vioxx to stop selling their product, although the FDA has done exhaustive evaluation of this pain reliever and says that the benefits outweigh the risks. The risk of more lawsuits is keeping a helpful medication from arthritis sufferers.

The one person who probably has the most influence in any lawsuit regarding the settlement and outcome of a case is the judge. Here is something to ponder. Should we have the right to vote for judges? Millions of dollars have been spent funding a campaign which encourages the appointment of judges over electing them. This is a hot topic in the legal community. Some people favor a system whereby judges are initially appointed and then must be re-elected to retain their seat, but others say the advantages of having judges answer to the public outweigh the disadvantages in all cases.

We all talk about frivolous lawsuits and laugh at the outrageous ones. Judges ultimately have the power to do something about them. As frivolous lawsuits earn larger settlements and more favorable decisions for plaintiffs, greed is encouraged and thrives and we all lose out. In West Virginia recently, the county school officials decided to remove all swing sets because of a few claims they have had to pay due to being sued by parents for a child's injury. So, all children will lose out on the fun of playing on the swings because a few greedy parents chose to sue. All sports equipment and sporting activities involve some risk of injury. Unless the injury is specifically due to a proven fault of the equipment, shouldn't the player realize that his/her action might cause an injury due simply to their choice to participate in the sport? Their choice should not create justification to later seek to find a way to be paid for their injury. It is truly sad that people are losing their sense of personal responsibility and a shame that people no longer want to accept the fact that accidents happen and that not every accident is someone else's fault. At what point did children and parents become absolved of any personal responsibility for their actions? When a parent sues the city because their child had a bike accident while riding on city sidewalks, will the county officials possibly decide to remove all sidewalks? There will be no end to ridiculous suits and insane monetary settlements until people make the choice to accept personal responsibility for their own actions in injury cases and stop blaming other people and parties for everything which happens to them. Your choice will matter.

CHOICES IN EDUCATION

Do you remember this song? School Days, school days, dear old golden rule days. Reading, and 'riting and 'rithmetic, taught to the tune of a hickory stick. You were my queen in calico, I was your barefoot, bashful beau. You wrote on my slate, "I love you so", when we were a couple of kids.

Oops, wait a minute. No hickory stick nowadays. That would be corporal punishment. Come to think of it, no good old golden rule days either. That could be religious. After all, the Golden Rule is in the Bible. A girl in calico? It's jeans and short skirts, and no beaus are bashful and bare-foot - they drive cars and wear Nike's. No slates either. It is computers in this day and age. A girl and a boy may still be a couple of kids, but they are a lot more worldly than we were as kids.

The schools are as different today as are the kids. I sym-pathize with the teachers who have to put up with unruly kids who disrupt their classrooms with impunity knowing that their parents will take the child's side over the teacher's no matter what. That is not to say that there are no bad teachers. There are some bad teachers and, unfortunately, they are protected by their unions or a tenure system which has outlived its usefulness.

Our old high school in Chicago now has metal detectors and a policeman on duty. I recently went to have lunch with my ten year old granddaughter at her school. The school was modern enough, but it was almost prison-like. Once in, the students could not leave and to get in it seemed as though I had to do everything but get fingerprinted. I think it is a sad commentary on our current society that our children are considered to be in such danger.

In my opinion, one of the biggest problems with our elementary and secondary schools is not the students, teachers or buildings. I think school administrators and school boards are generally way off base. Our news is rife with examples of school administrations making dumb decisions. It seems they are always enforcing rules to ridiculous extremes without using any common sense. They hyperventilate if a girl brings an aspirin to school or a boy innocently includes a fork and a dull knife in his lunch box. Also, there was a time not that long ago when positions on the local school board were voluntary and dedicated citizens served without pay. Now, the school board members might make as much as the teachers. Not a good idea.

In spite of the fact that our country spends more per pupil than most other developed nations, the statistics are pretty bleak. In the past 30 years, we have fallen from 1st place in high school and college graduation rates to 18th place. Our 15 year olds now rank 25th internationally in math, 21st in science, 15th in reading literacy and 24th in problem solving skills.

However, with all the perceived problems, our public

educational system still chugs along pretty well. It is so easy to criticize and forget the obstacles faced by the public schools today. These obstacles include deteriorating study habits in the home (due to broken families, too much TV, pockets of poverty, lax parental supervision and guidance), the need to accommodate children with physical and emotional disabilities, teen-age mothers, an alarming number of children being diagnosed with Attention Deficit Disorder (ADD), autistic children, too many planned extra-curricular activities etc...

The two hot-button emotional issues in education today are prayer in schools and vouchers. These two issues have moved into the political realm. Conservatives generally choose to believe that prayer in the schools and vouchers for private schools are good. Liberals generally chose to think that prayer in schools and school vouchers are not good. Independents have to decide between the two choices.

When we speak of prayer in school, we must realize that this is not a discussion about private schools. Most private schools are religious in nature and public funds are not involved. Thus, if a private school wants to require that its pupils pray to or through God, Allah, Moses, Mary, Jesus or the man on the moon, that is their choice and it is the choice of the parents, who are footing the bill. It gets sticky when it comes to taxpayer supported public schools. Religiously conservative friends have told us how terrible it is that the Supreme Court has taken God out of the schools and forbidden children from praying in school. We think that they are wrong. We attended Chicago public schools and were never aware that God was in our schools. Also, we never had teachers leading us in prayers in school. We don't feel that the lack of school prayer damaged us in any way.

What is important to remember in the public school prayer debate is that the Supreme Court did not outlaw prayer in schools, it only forbid teacher-led or formal school prayers. All students may discretely pray in schools. The courts did not say that when a student was confronted with a pop quiz, he or she could not silently offer up a prayer for help. Most people who support school or teacher-led prayer in public schools are thinking of "their" kind of prayer. How comfortable would a Protestant Christian be with a prayer asking for intervention by the Virgin Mary, a Jew being asked to pray in the name of Jesus, or a Christian or Jew being asked in a prayer to bow down to Allah? We choose to believe that any prayer in taxpayer funded public schools should not be official, but a private matter. It may be true that the Supreme Court went too far when it ruled against official moments of silent prayer in classrooms, but we can live with that.

Vouchers are even a bigger issue than school prayer. Voucher supporters want the government to give them a voucher which can be used to pay for the expenses they incur in sending their children to private schools. They point out that they are forced to pay taxes to support public education and want the opportunity to send their children to an elite private or religious school, rather than a public school. On the surface, this sounds like a reasonable argument, but it really is not.

Voucher supporters can send their children to private or religious schools now - many of them do. Their problem is that they must pay extra for that choice. That is the way it is with public services, be they education (public versus private schools), transportation (public buses versus private cars or taxis), sports (municipal tennis courts versus a private tennis club), and so on. I can see wealthy people, who send their children to an elite private academy, subsidizing poorer people by paying their share of public school taxes, even if they do not choose to use those public schools. I have difficulty seeing how we can ask poorer people to subsidize the wealthy by paying for their private school expenses.

Proponents of vouchers say:

1. With vouchers, poor people can get a wider choice.
2. Vouchers promote free market competition between public and private schools.
3. There should be no public schools, just private schools with vouchers.
4. Students do better in private schools.
5. Vouchers give parents more freedom.
6. Private schools (especially religious) cost less to operate.

Opponents of Vouchers say:

1. Vouchers would drain funding from public schools.
2. Private schools practice cream skimming (selecting only students who belong to a preferred economic, religious, or ethnic group).

3. Private schools cost less to operate because public schools take children with behavioral, physical, and emotional problems.
4. Public schools are accountable to taxpayers, private schools are not, but would use public funds.
5. Vouchers would cost taxpayers more.
6. Government money should not be used for teaching religion.

Most of the private school enrollment in this country is in religious schools. There are many parents who presently send their children to religious schools or would like to do so. We feel that the most important question about vouchers is, should our government pay for a student's religious education?

Paul:
    A few years ago, my granddaughter, who attended a private Christian elementary school, had a part in a performance at her school. I, as a devoted grandparent, went kicking and screaming to the event. The program began with the "Pledge of Allegiance" to the U.S. flag. Great! Our country is a wonderful place and I feel that the "Pledge of Allegiance" is appropriate for kids and adults too. Also, having "under God" in it does not bother me a bit. I rather like it. After that pledge, they had a pledge to the Christian flag. I don't know where the Christian flag came from, but sure enough, when I

looked closely I saw another flag next to the U.S. flag. I guess that was the Christian flag. The third pledge was a pledge of allegiance to the Bible. Although I am a Christian, I had never heard of a pledge of allegiance to the Christian flag or the Bible before. I guess that it is O.K. and I can believe that my granddaughter may experience positive religious or moral growth through saying these pledges. I think that it is fair to assume that these pledges set the tone for the rest of her educational experience at this school. Regardless of what a great thing this may be, I ask myself the question: Should people of a different religious persuasion be required to pay for the Christian education of my granddaughter? I do not think so.

Choice in education is presently available without vouchers. Private schooling results in extra cost. It is rather like playing tennis on the free municipal courts versus joining a private tennis club. As a society, we can chose to spend our public funds to fund private schools through the voucher system, or we can let those who decide to chose a special extra-fee school pay for that privilege themselves. We do not feel that it is right to support any private schools, especially religious schools (even Christian) through public tax dollars. This issue will be decided through our political system. Vote for your choice!

LABELS OF
CHOICE

So far, the choices we have discussed are independent of each other. The choice to use or not use certain drugs is not connected to a choice we might make in our end of life situation. Our choice regarding whether or not to support women's reproductive rights is separate from the position we might choose in dealing with the questions of population control, health care, etc. There is, however, one choice we have to make which has a direct effect on our ability to make all of these other choices in our lives. That choice is in the area of politics, and no matter how we feel about it, the politicians we support, when elected, very definitely have a large measure of control over whether or not we will have individual free choice in the matters which have been addressed in this book.

In the U.S. today, we are faced with choosing to be a Republican, Democrat, or Independent and accepting a conservative or liberal (some say "progressive") philosophy. It seems like it should be an easy choice to make, but it is not. It is confusing because the political parties are not always what they seem to be and their political philosophies have become blurred over the years.

When the U.S. was founded, it was the liberals who generally favored individual rights and freedoms and opposed a strong centralized government. In fact, the Latin word "liber" means free. The concept of individual rights and freedoms was never codified until the revolution and the forming of our government. The modern Democrat party likes to harken back to Thomas Jefferson as its founder. He and his followers were in favor of states rights and feared too strong a central government. The Republicans did not exist at that time, but the conservatives of that era favored the status quo and a stronger centralized government. Those positions were championed by the monarchists during the revolution and later by Alexander Hamilton and the Federalists.

The Republicans refer back to Abraham Lincoln as the founder of their party. They frequently call themselves, "The Party of Lincoln". Today, the Republican party unabashedly claims to be conservative, favors the status quo, and has a definite "rightward slant". But, during the Civil War time, the era of its founder Abraham Lincoln, the Republican Party created major social change with the adoption of the 13th, 14th, and 15th amendments and it adopted our country's first individual income tax. This tax was passed in 1862 to finance the war and existed for ten years. With the end of the Civil War and passing of the 13th, 14th, and 15th amendments, the whites in the south became almost exclusively Democrats (southern Democrats to be sure). After the 1964 Civil Rights Act, which was passed by the Democrats, most of the white southern Democrats then switched to the Republican party, where many of them remain today - a sad vestige of latent racism.

Today's political parties, Democrat and Republican, are not what they were historically. The Democrat party is not the small government party of its founders at the beginning of our republic. Today's Democrat party draws its support from the masses and argues that government should be a strong force for social change, help the disadvantaged in our society, and protect the individual rights of all Americans. It derives much of its support from unions and minority groups. As a party, it argues that the government should guarantee that everyone should have affordable access to quality education and health care.

The Republican party is not the party of change it was in its formative years either. Today's Republican party attracts pro-gun supporters (who feel they need weapons for hunting, protecting their home and family, and in possible defense against an attack on our country), business corporations (especially the defense and health care industries, and the Chamber of Commerce) who want less government regulation and fewer environmental restrictions. Republicans also attract wealthier citizens who feel they benefit from limiting various social programs and reducing taxes, and the conservative fundamentalist religious groups, who are concerned about social/religious matters and want to incorporate those concerns into society.

It is important to recognize that both of our political parties exist only to install their people into positions of power and authority in our government. To do this, they troll for support among the electorate by stirring up passions and fever over issues such as the economy, national security, the environment, government influence in our lives, and matters of social or moral conscience. Frequently they use a variety of wedge issues. They claim to be philosophically faithful to their positions, but that is not entirely true. Today, liberals want more individual freedoms in social areas such as free speech and sexual matters, and more restrictions on business and environmental matters. Conservatives want to emphasize individual freedom in non-social issues such as less regulation of business and want more restrictions in social matters. The difference between change and the status quo is still with us, but how it applies depends upon the issue. We have a case of situational philosophy. For example, the Republican party says it wants less government in our lives, but believes government should dictate the most personal issue of women's reproductive rights. The Democrat party believes government should help our blue collar workers, but favors blanket amnesty for illegal immigrants which will reduce employment opportunities for our home-grown workers. Both parties are against deficit spending, unless they are in power and can direct that spending to their supporters or further their own philosophical goals. It is interesting to note that a liberal in Texas is not the same as a liberal in New York and a conservative in Oregon is not the same as a conservative in South Carolina. The liberal/conservative labels are not so rigid today. Consider, for instance, the case of Barry Goldwater. He was Mr. Conservative in 1964. He was against prolific government spending, but was pro-choice and favored some forms of gun control. Or consider John F. Kennedy, who drastically lowered taxes while he was president. How would their opinions fare in their political parties today?

We believe that when we support a candidate for office with our vote, that vote should be based upon whether that candidate, if elected, will uphold our right to freely make the individual choices which are important to us and who will be guided by some of our personal views as described in this book.

IS THERE A STATESMAN IN THE HOUSE?

"What, no television"? Those were the words gasped by our 4 and 7 year old granddaughters in June of 2004. We had taken "the girls" to spend a month with us in our newly purchased summer place in the North Carolina mountains. It was an election year and the television sets were bursting with political ads, the vast majority of which featured either cruel negative attacks and ugly un-substantiated charges against opponents or preposterous claims and righteous indignation preached on behalf of candidates, many of whom were mediocre at best. The cable television talk shows had degenerated into shouting matches where partisan talking heads interrupted each other constantly and mouthed slogans and talking points of the day.

It was in this environment that we said, "Enough", and decided not to hook up the cable for that summer. We would read books instead. Our granddaughters were hor-rified at the prospect of one month without television. We did question the sanity of our decision, but it worked out well. Our granddaughters learned to play outside, on their own, without adults breathing down their necks and we read a lot of books and played games with our girls.

None of us missed seeing the political mumbo-jumbo which seemed to have taken over the tube.

Our negative reaction to television political advertising and talk shows may have been extreme, but it does illustrate how aggravating the political stridency can be, especially during an election year. Toss in robo calls and it is difficult to escape. Unfortunately, if we choose to live in a politically free society, we have to accept the bad along with the good. The good is that we have free speech which allows us to hear differing points of view and different arguments before choosing how to vote. But what do we hear? Sometimes we hear common sense and verifiable facts woven into rational arguments which will aid us in choosing to make good political decisions. More often, we hear falsehoods and half-truths repeated over and over. If a lie is repeated enough times, many people will start to believe it. For example, a poll in August of 2010 showed that 18% of those polled believed that President Obama is a Muslim, yet there is no factual basis for that belief. It has been disproved again and again, but the claim has been made over and over on the internet, by conservative talk show personalities, and politicians, so that some people believe it regardless of the evidence. Another example is the statement by dear friends of ours who believe it is very possible that President Obama was not born in the United States and was, therefore, not eligible to be president of the U.S.. They told us they held that opinion because a friend of theirs, a retired judge whom they respected, held that belief. When we expressed our surprise at that belief, our friends defended their position by saying that they had not personally seen a birth certificate (even though copies of Obama's birth certificate have been published and attested to by numerous reporters and government officials). The erroneous "birther" controversy has, like the Obama religious fantasy, been repeated enough times by rumor mongers that some people believe it, regardless of the facts.

We need to choose carefully when we make our political decisions. We need to remember, as discussed in the prior chapter, that, "Both of our political parties exist only to install their people into positions of political power and authority in our government". They stir up passions and fever over issues to obtain that end. In making our choices, we need to separate facts from fiction. This leads us back to the television political advertising situation. Much of the negative political advertising is paid for by so called "independent" groups rather than the candidates themselves. Sad to say, misleading negative advertising works, especially if repeated often enough. Candidates do not like to run negative ads themselves, so they rely on the "independent" groups to do it for them. More and more often these groups are set up as non-profit organizations. As such, they do not have to disclose their donors. This means that the public really has no idea who is bankrolling these negative ads. Total spending on congressional elections in non-presidential years has more than doubled in the past twelve years. In the 2010 election, it almost reached four billion dollars.

The Supreme Court ruling in 2010 gave corporations and labor unions the right to spend unlimited amounts to back or attack individual candidates. This striking down of limits on the size of union and corporate political contributions has opened the floodgates and accounts for much of the 2010 increase in political spending. Arguments can be made supporting or condemning this Supreme Court decision but, in all probability, little can be done to change it. Laws requiring not-for-profit organizations to disclose their donors would at least allow the public to see who is paying for these ads. Federal legislation requiring disclosure was introduced in 2010. It was called The Disclosure Act, but it went nowhere. Democrats in the House of Representatives ruined the House version by allowing exemptions for powerful special interest groups, such as AARP, The Sierra Club, and the National Rifle Association. The Republicans filibustered the act in the Senate. Until this situation is corrected, we need to exercise caution in heeding negative ads underwritten by shadowy groups when making our political choices. In the meantime, should we not encourage our lawmakers to act like statesmen, take the risk of anonymous attacks from special interests, and require donor exposure?

In the previous paragraph, we refer to statesmen, rather than politicians. There is a difference between the two. Webster's dictionary refers to a statesman and a politician as people versed in the principles of government and engaging in the business of government or shaping its policies. He then proceeds to differentiate between the two, by explaining that a statesman exercises political leadership wisely and without narrow partisanship, while a politician is a person engaged in party politics as a profession - a person primarily interested in political office for selfish or other usually short-sighted reasons.

Assuming Webster's definitions to be correct, it is clear we have far more politicians than statesmen in Congress today. Political polarization in Washington D.C. has reached an extraordinary level. The political center has all but disappeared. There are a few moderate Democrats (known as Blue Dogs) but that is about it. For the most part, the more moderate Democrats and Republicans have been defeated in their primaries or withered away. In the past, these centrist Republicans and Democrats were able to set aside extreme views and work together to get things done. Today, the Senate has become a dysfunctional body rather than a deliberative one. The use of the filibuster, once rare, has become routine. Huge amounts of money flow into election campaigns. The need for this money for re-election purposes makes these professional politicians all the more susceptible to supporting narrow policies of special interest groups contributing legal bribes, rather than supporting policies in the public interest or good for the nation as a whole.

The cash received from and subsequent favors given to special interest groups in order to get elected and be re-elected will continue unabated. In the current political climate, if a candidate does not play the money game and become a pawn of the special interest masters, the candidate needs to be super wealthy to self-finance a good portion of his or her campaign. Self financing of political campaigns is becoming more common. One of the candidates in 2010 for the governor of California is said to have spent over one hundred million dollars of her own money - to secure a job which pays $212,000 a year. A 2010 Senate candidate in Wisconsin reportedly has spent 4.5 million dollars to gain a position which pays $193,000 a year. Why? Maybe they want to be a statesman. Maybe it is an ego trip. Perhaps they are frustrated by our present government and feel that they can make better decisions. They can spend their money as they wish.

Many people feel that money is having too great an influence in our government. Perhaps it has always been that way. As a free society, however, we should be able to choose to limit the excessive influence created by special interest money. The imposition of term limits and the availability of a better public election financing program would go far towards weakening special interests. The choice to impose such limits lies with the voters. In the meantime, we need to examine the source of the political material before us, cut out the chaff, and make a careful attempt to vote for statesmen. In our opinion, the ideal society would have a government which would provide for the maximum individual freedom possible consistent with a just and orderly society. That would require electing statesmen, not politicians.

WAR V.
PEACE

I am amazed at the American public's docile acceptance of our government's continued engagement in a seven year war and a nine year war. They have been fought at the same time in two backward countries which have about as much chance of overcoming tribal and religious differences and establishing modern free, democratic societies as they do of colonizing the moon. As I think more about this, I come to realize that, contrary to what the average American probably thinks, we have become a pretty militaristic nation. Prior to the year of my birth (1935) I figure that our country was at war for eighteen out of one hundred and fifty-nine years, about 11% of the time. That calculation includes our War of Independence and the Civil War, but not the continuing pacification of the native Americans. That changed with WWII and during my lifetime we have been at war about 40% of the time and that does not include short skirmishes in Beirut, Panama, Grenada, Somalia, and Yugoslavia.

What has caused this (apparent) increase in militarism? There could be a number of peripheral reasons, but I think that the main reason is a realignment of power within the U.S. itself. Until WWII, the U.S. had no permanent armaments industry. Prior to that time, we adjusted peacetime production to war-time production and then switched back to primarily peacetime production when the conflict ended. This changed in WWII when a more permanent armaments industry was established.

President Eisenhower addressed this change in his farewell address to the nation on January 17, 1961. He said, "The conjunction of an immense military establishment and a large arms industry is new in the American experience". Ike recognized the need for this development, but warned of its grave complications. He further said, "We must never let the weight of this combination endanger our liberties or democratic processes".

Was Eisenhower right when he issued those warnings? Have we adequately guarded against unwarranted influence of the military industrial complex? Is there a military industrial complex? In 2009, the military budget was 651.2 billion dollars. When off-budget items are included, the amount is about 20% of our governments total expenditures. We officially have 737 military bases in 130 countries outside of the United States. However, the unofficial true number is estimated as being over 1,000 since there are many bases which are secret or classified for "security reasons". Consider this. We still have 268 bases in Germany and 127 bases in Japan and WWII ended 65 years ago.

Before we disregard President Eisenhower's warning about never letting, "The weight of this combination endanger our liberties or democracy", we should remember that in his farewell speech he further warned about making sweeping transformations to American life on the basis of national security. In the past ten years, we have seen our government suspend habeas corpus for some American citizens and engage in secret interceptions of personal emails and telephone conversations without judicial approval in the name of "national security". I can't help but think of George Orwell's book entitled "1984". It concerns a country in a perpetual state of war and with pervasive government surveillance. It was this book which introduced the term "Big Brother" to us. Is fiction becoming reality?

Eisenhower said there has to be balance in just about everything. The lobbying power of the permanent industrial military complex and seemingly permanent professional military establishment has thrown us out of balance. War is profitable so, unfortunately, we will probably see more of it.

Paul:
I don't know about you, but I am tired of war. I realize the fact that I wore a U.S. Army uniform for three years neither makes me a hero nor an expert in world affairs. I realize there are evil people in the world who envy us and hate us and we must protect ourselves from these monsters. But 20% of every dollar spent for defense? One thousand military bases on foreign soil? Giving up constitutional rights in the name of national security? When "Big Brother" can take away the right of habeas corpus from our neighbor, he can take it away from us. When "Big Brother" can secretly monitor our neighbors

telephone calls or investigate their library records, he can do the same to us.

It seems sad to me that we, as a nation, seem unable to overcome our fears and the influence of the military industrial complex. We should be able to say, "End these two current military excursions, NOW", "Get rid of most of those 1,000 bases on foreign soil", "Stop being the world's policeman and protect our borders", and "Spend the money saved by reducing our deficit or providing our citizens with a plan for decent health care". I don't think that I am being unpatriotic to say that I am tired of war and fed up with spending huge sums of money, as well as our blood, in foreign lands. It is my opinion that by occupying Iraq and Afghanistan we are only fueling more hatred towards us and creating more willing terrorists.

A task force commissioned by Defense Secretary Donald Rumsfeld in 2004 concluded that "Muslims do not 'hate our freedom', but rather, they hate our policies", such as, American direct intervention in the Muslim world, through our one-sided support in favor of Israel, support for Islamic tyrannies in places like Egypt and Saudi Arabia, and, most of all, the American occupation of Iraq and Afghanistan. A more recent study by Prof. Robert Pate, a University of Chicago political science professor, confirms the Defense Department study: namely, that the prime cause of terrorist suicide bombings is not Hatred of our Freedoms, Inherent Violence in Islamic Culture, or a Desire for Worldwide Sharia Rule by Caliphate. Instead the prime cause is foreign military occupations. Pape said, "…we have lots of evidence now that when you put the foreign military presence in, it triggers suicide terrorism campaigns,…and that when the foreign forces leave, it takes away almost 100% of the terrorist campaign". There was a spike in suicide bombings in Afghanistan after we expanded our presence in 2006 and again in 2010.

In his farewell speech, President Eisenhower also said, "Only an alert and knowledgeable citizenry can compel the proper meshing of the huge industrial and military machinery of defense with our peaceful methods and goals, so that security and liberty may prosper together". The choice is ours to make.

POPULATION

Twenty years ago a group called "Negative Population Growth" compiled and published a book of scholarly papers called "The Case For Fewer People". It addressed population problems facing the U.S. and the world. Some of the statistics from these papers are incorporated in this chapter addressing population problems. It has long been our feeling that most of our environmental problems in the U.S. and the world are exacerbated by our burgeoning populations. Yet, when the problems of deteriorating air and water quality, garbage disposal, loss of forests and accompanying erosion, slums and related crime are addressed by our government, the answers which they proffer never address the main reason - too many people. There are already too many people in the U.S. to provide for the sustainability of our natural resources. The projected increase in the population of third world countries, which already have abysmally low living standards, will continue to affect us in the United States. The effect of third world poverty is putting pressure on our fragile economic situation. There are twelve plus million illegals who have poured into our country trying to escape crowding and poverty. From 1990 to 2000 the projected population increase in third world countries was over 800 million and has not slowed down. We are already overcrowded in the U.S. and have our own problems of over-population to face. We can not take in over a billion and a half under-educated people just because they are starving. It is high time that our government faces up to our over-population and illegal immigration problems. We, because of our own over-population problems, can no longer be the country of, "Give me your tired, your poor". We can not afford it!

Giving aid to countries wanting assistance in limiting human fertility should be our contribution to third world countries - not taking them all in. Mexico made a decision in the 70's to bring down its very high birth rate and has implemented programs which have brought the total fertility rate down from 6.7 to 3.7. That, alone, reduced their 2000 projected population by almost thirty million. Central America has not fared as well as Mexico in bringing their fertility rate down. They have encountered strong religious objections to family planning and contraceptives, causing living conditions to fall back to 1960 levels. With population momentum still over the sustaining rate, neither Central America nor Mexico is likely to stabilize their population in time to prevent severe stress on their ecological, social, and economic systems which will, in turn, affect ours.

As previously pointed out when discussing jobs, illegal immigration must be halted. If not, many of our under-educated citizens, black, white, and Hispanic will be unable to find jobs and will continue to be socially marginalized. The last thing our under-educated need is more competition from immigrants for the limited number of jobs available to them or more competition in seeking the education needed to obtain better jobs. Some legal immigration of educated people is advantageous because we, as a nation, are not producing students with adequate educational preparation in certain sectors. Often over-population concerns are dismissed with the argument that our percentage of immigrants to citizens today is lower than in 1910. More faulty reasoning, based on the absurdity that the U.S. should continue to grow at a rate which was acceptable during the industrial revolution. Times have changed and our needs have changed from a country which had lots of jobs and opportunities for a growing population to a country not having enough jobs for its too-large population. Another dismissal of the problems of over-population comes from the "Right Camp" with their label of "Demographic Winter" describing their "birth dearth" concept. They claim that declining birthrates among white people in the U.S. and Europe will lead to the end of Western Civilization as we know it, along with all sorts of catastrophic events. While it is true that there are higher rates of births among non-whites, that, in itself, is no reason to add to our over-crowded world by encouraging a "Fair-skinned Fertility Fest" with "prizes for pregnancies".

One important factor which affects our over-population is the misinterpretation of the 14th amendment. When you were a child, I'm sure that you often heard the old adage, "Two wrongs don't make a right". Well, in the case of "anchor babies" that doesn't seem to be true. What is an "anchor baby"? It is the product of a new attitude, "Two wrongs do make a right". Under our present legal interpretation, an "anchor baby", the baby of illegal parents, becomes an American citizen if it is born in the U.S. These children may instantly qualify for welfare. In addition, with the passage of the 1965 Immigration and Nationality Act, the child may, at the age of 21, sponsor other family members for entry into the U.S. The prospects and numbers involved are staggering, especially when you consider that in two hospitals, one in California and one in Texas, 70% of the babies born in one year were "anchor babies". The cost for 11,200 of those babies was as follows: $34.5 million to deliver them, $9.5 million in federal aid, and another $31.3 million from the local governments. The 14th amendment, ratified to ensure citizenship for newly-freed slaves, extended to, " All persons, born or naturalized in the United States and subject to the jurisdiction thereof". The phrase, "Subject to the jurisdiction thereof", excluded Native Americans because of their tribal jurisdiction, as well as foreign visitors, ambassadors and their babies born here. In the case of illegal aliens, their native country has a claim of allegiance on the child. Why then, are "anchor babies" being given immediate citizenship and benefits? This is wrong!

Schools also bear a burden regarding these "anchor babies" of illegals. With estimates of 425,000 children being born to people illegally in our country each year, the tax burden on every citizen to educate these children is high and unfair. The original intent of the 14th amendment was certainly not to make it easy for illegals to get citizenship for their babies at the cost of each tax-paying citizen. This situation is ludicrous! The U.S. must, like most other developed countries, correct this problem by having the Congress adopt legislation which will clarify the 14th amendment to specifically not include the children of those who have defied our laws by sneaking into our country. Only three factors determine population size. Mortality is untouchable because we all advocate longevity. Fertility is another, and while declines should be encouraged, they are not enforceable. The last, immigration, is the most obvious factor. Even the clarification of the 14th amendment now and deportation of all illegals (with their "anchor babies") will leave millions of "anchor babies" to return when they turn twenty-one and are able to sponsor their families. We must stop this stupid misinterpretation of the 14th amendment - now!

What is the optimal figure for population in the U.S.? - the world? There seems to be a built-in desire for growth among Americans with Texans striving to pass up New Yorkers as California did in 1963. City dwellers are happy when their city population surpasses that of comparable cities. That type of thinking must end. We think that we need to take into consideration that in 1995 some experts came up with the optimal figure for our country to be one hundred million. That figure was based on our being self-sustaining in solar energy and also on our land, water, and biological resources. That figure was far below the two hundred forty-six million we had at that time. Though that figure may be low, it points out the dire need to limit the two variable factors we can - the factor of immigration in the U.S. and fertility both in the U.S. and the world. The conclusion which the UN Conference on Population and Development should have made in 1994, but didn't, would have been a strategy for a global effort to reduce the world fertility rate to replacement level by 2010 - today. Such an endeavor would have been the best chance we have to stabilize the world's population at less than ten billion by the end of this century. Our ability to do this will critically determine the future of humanity. Not only was no strategy for implementation adopted but, "Right Camp" administrations in our country even cut out 34 million in aid per year to third world countries to help with family planning even when that aid money did not fund any abortions.

Instead of moving forward in the past sixteen years towards population reduction, we have made little or no progress. We must immediately begin to make family planning available to those who wish to have fewer children, but lack the means or money to do so. Secondly, we must develop individual and community incentives which create a desire to have no more than two children per family. A possible global population between twelve and seventeen billion by the year 2100 (doubling from six billion today) will result in a great loss of human dignity, increased mortality, drastic pollution and other environmental changes, and the extinction of species. How can we achieve the goal of dropping fertility rates to replacement rates? "Right Camp" moral objections must be overcome. Hopefully, they can be convinced that, through contraception and education, abortion rates can be lowered, as well as infant and maternal mortality rates. No one should object to those goals. However, women's choices in these private matters must not be restricted. State and community incentives can point out the advantages of a small family and encourage small families by reducing the perceived need for large families to provide economic security. Other incentives might be benefits for small families in areas of jobs, education and reduction of taxes.

Over-population can not dignify anyone. It is at odds with the value of every human being. The "Right Camp" mantra, "sanctity of life" is at the opposite end of the spectrum from the apocalyptic human suffering which will be the outcome of unchecked population. The perceived value of every human person suffers in a world with too many people.

It is always a good policy to wrap one's proposals and arguments with such words as: "fair", "moral", "ethical", and "just", etc. We hope that we have presented most of our ideas fairly. No doubt, our personal feelings have colored our choice of wording and characterization at times, but the frustrations we have felt on so many issues have born this book, such as it is. Some of our ideas may be called "nutty" or be viewed as draconian, but all of our ideas are just that - ideas. The choice to consider them and/or act on them is yours and, CHOICE MATTERS.

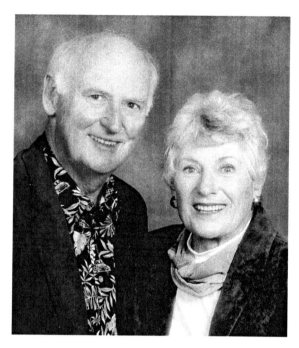

About the Authors

Barbara and Paul Gerhardt are the co-authors of "Choice Matters". Born and raised in Chicago, they both attended the University of Colorado. Paul served for thirty years as the executive director of the American Accounting Association. "Choice Matters" is his second book. His first book was a humorous novel entitled "Feline Four", filled with twists and turns.

Barbara worked in real estate sales and as a property manager. In addition she has written and illustrated two children's books. The first, "I AM of Scram" was published in 2007. Her second book, "Pathways" provides a delightful trip to the zoo with whimsical rhyme and pictures for grandparents, parents and young children.

The Gerhardt's have lived in Sarasota, Florida for the past 39 years, during which time they have hashed and re-hashed the questions and concerns which provide the basis for "Choice Matters". Their book seeks to stimulate thought and discussion on a myriad of issues and illustrate the importance of well-thought out, pragmatic choice in our personal and public life.

LaVergne, TN USA
03 April 2011
222643LV00003B/1/P

9 781936 343577